Christian Character, Virtue, and Bioethics

Proceedings of the 1996
Clinical Bioethics Conference

June 27–29, 1996
Vancouver, British Columbia

Sponsored by:
Christian Medical Dental Society of Canada
and Regent College

Dr. Edwin C. Hui, Editor

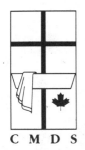

C M D S

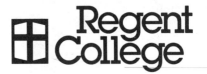

First published by Regent College, 1996
5800 University Boulevard, Vancouver, B.C. V6T 2E4 Canada
(604) 224-3245

Typesetting by Paul Chapman
Cover design by Irma J. Bennett and Dal Schindell

Printed in Canada

ISBN 1-57383-067-4

Contents

Part III: Virtue of Love

Introduction

Twentieth-century medicine has been characterized by very sophisticated and useful technologies; but it has accomplished this at a cost of losing the patient as a person in the midst of all the "high tech" equipments. Similarly, twentieth-century moral philosophy has developed a set of bioethical principles which often provide useful guidelines in solving medico-ethical dilemmas, but suffer from being abstracted formulations remote from the various clinical contexts. In short, modern medicine suffers from the loss of the authentic personal relationships crucial in medicine and medical care.

The second Christian Bioethics Conference, jointly sponsored by Regent College and the Christian Medical Dental Society of Canada, was held in Vancouver, B.C., on June 27-29, 1996. The Conference was entitled "Christian Character, Virtue, and Bioethics," and a panel of seventeen theologians, philosophers, and clinicians were invited to speak on various subjects seeking to recover the importance of the relational dimension intrinsic to the clinical encounter between the health care provider and the patient. More specifically, the presentations were focused on how the Christian virtues of faith, hope, and love have provided the foundation for Christian character vital to the sustenance of such relationships. This volume contains the proceedings of this three-day conference.

Dr. J. I. Packer opened the conference with a keynote address on the theological virtue of faith which provides a covenantal foundation for the relationship between health care providers and recipients. This theological exposition was followed by three presentations dealing with the issues of money, power, and sex in the medical profession: "A Christian Ethic of Financing Health Care and Physicians' Income" by Dr. John Hux; "The Power of the Physician: A Christian

Perspective" by Drs. Arthur Froese, Sheldene Simola, and Kevin Parker; and "Chastity in the Practice of Medicine" by Fr. Dr. Joseph Soria. Dr. David Neima ended the day with a meditation on Pope John Paul II's *Evangelium vitae*.

The theological virtue of hope was expounded by Dr. Edwin Hui in a context of patient care and the development of medical technology, which have recently been guided by a secularized version of hope instead of an authentic Christian eschatology. This was followed by three essays: "When Is Enough, Enough?" by Dr. Robert Stephens; "Advance Directives: A Christian Appraisal" by Dr. John Senn; and "The Technological Evolution of Reproduction" by Dr. Stephen Genuis. The second day was concluded by an exposition of the "Beatitudes as a Basis for Medical Ethics" by Dr. John Patrick.

A theological commentary on the virtue of love was provided by Dr. Stanley Grenz whose essay suggests how *agape* may be integrated in *filial* friendship, marital, and medical relationships. This theme was further illustrated by a number of essays: "Care, a Basis of Physician-Patient Relationship: 'Who Is My Brother?'" by Dr. Margaret Cottle; "Sexuality in the 1990s" by Dr. Stephen Genuis; and "Quality of Life, Christian Love, and Sanctity of Life" by Dr. Sheila Harding. Three special seminars were given on the subjects of "Contraception," "Natural Family Planning," and "Christian Character and Professionalism" by Dr. Agnes Tanguay, Dr. Howard Bright, and Dr. J. Gerald Higgins respectively. The conference was concluded by a time of prayer and a homily entitled "These Three Remain: Faith, Hope, Love" delivered by Dr. James Houston.

I would like to thank all keynote and plenary speakers for their effort in making the presentations and contributing to this volume. Special appreciation goes to Drs. Robert O. Stephens, David Neima, Sherif S. Hanna, and Sheila Harding for their suggestions and participation in the design of the conference. Thanks also go to Dal Schindell, Irma J. Bennett, Paul Chapman, Jane Rowland, and Tatchi Yuen for their able help in the copy editing, proof-reading, typesetting, and publication of the proceedings.

Edwin C. Hui, MD, PhD, Editor
Regent College, Vancouver, B.C.
July 1996

Authors

Dr. Howie Bright
: Clinical Instructor for Family Practice, University of British Columbia; Local Medical Coordinator, B.C. Ambulance Service.

Dr. Margaret Cottle
: Palliative Care—visiting staff of Vancouver Hospital and Health Sciences Centre; Chair of Focus on the Family Physician Advisory Council.

Dr. Arthur Froese
: Associate Professor of Psychiatry and Paediatrics, Queens University, Kingston, Ont.; National Treasurer of CMDS Canada.

Dr. Stephen Genuis
: Associate Professor of Obstetrics and Gynaecology, University of Alberta; Member, Physicians Resource Council, Focus on the Family.

Dr. Stanley Grenz
: Pioneer McDonald Professor of Baptist Heritage, Theology, and Ethics, Carey Theological College.

Dr. Sheila Harding
: Associate Professor of Haematology, University of Saskatchewan; Assistant Director of Educational Support and Development in the College of Medicine; Chair of CMDS Ethics Committee.

Dr. Gerald Higgins
: Professor of Bioethics, University of Alberta; Formerly Chairman and Professor of Family Medicine, University of Alberta.

Dr. James Houston
: Board of Governors' Professor of Spiritual Theology, Regent College.

Dr. Edwin Hui
: Associate Professor of Medical Ethics, Spiritual Theology, and Chinese Studies, Regent College; Ethicist of the Ethics Advisory Council of British Columbia Cancer Agency.

Dr. Jan Hux
: Specialist in Internal Medicine; Staff mem-

	ber of Institute for Clinical Evaluative Sciences, Toronto.
Dr. David Neima	Ophthalmologist, New Westminster, B.C.; Past President of CMDS Canada.
Dr. J. I. Packer	Sangwoo Youtong Chee Professor of Theology, Regent College; Senior Editor and Visiting Scholar for *Christianity Today*.
Dr. John Patrick	Associate Professor of Biochemistry and Paediatrics, University of Ottawa; Coordinator of Field Ministries, CMDS Canada.
Dr. John Senn	Head of Clinical Haematology and Director of Clinical Ethics at Sunnybrook Health Sciences Centre, Toronto. Emeritus Professor, University of Toronto.
Fr. Joseph Soria, MD	Priest of Opus Dei, an Evangelical movement in the Catholic Church.
Dr. Robert Stephens	Family Physician; Executive Director CMDS Canada and Evangelical Medical Aid Society.
Dr. Arnold Voth	Assistant Clinical Professor of Internal Medicine, University of Alberta.

Part I

Virtue of Faith

J. I. Packer

Faith, Covenant, and Medical Practice

A sentence which, I confess, made me laugh when first I read it nearly fifty years ago, and which has always stuck in my mind because of its grotesque overtones, is the translation of the fifteenth verse of the thirty-eighth chapter of the apocryphal book Ecclesiasticus in the English Revised Version of 1884, which was the text from which in those days Oxford's theological students were required to work. The RV renders the verse as follows: "He that sinneth before his Maker, let him fall into the hands of the physician." That sounds awful, as if coming under medical care is a fitting judgment from God on impiety and is one of the worst things that can happen to you. However, that is not what is meant; the thought that the Greek text of Ecclesiasticus is expressing is simply that illness as such would be a just judgment from God on deliberate sin. And in any case the Greek translation of ben-Sirach's Hebrew, which the RV followed, seems to miss the meaning of the original; thus the NRSV of 1989 renders the verse as follows: "He who sins against his Maker, will be defiant toward the physician"—the point being that one whose life-strategy is rebellion against God is likely to prove a self-willed, obstreperous patient. This, which seems to be the true sense of the words, is probably not news to any single one of us, and it might indeed relieve some of our personal and professional desperations when we realize that this insight goes back at least to the second century before Christ.

The verse is actually rounding off a passage in which the writer celebrates God's gift to mankind of medical science and medical personnel. I would like you to hear some of the things that he says about this matter.

Honour physicians for their services,
  for the Lord created them;
for their gift of healing comes from the Most High,
  and they are rewarded by the king.
The skill of physicians makes them distinguished,
  and in the presence of the great they are admired.
The Lord created medicines out of the earth,
  and the sensible will not despise them. . . .

My child, when you are ill, do not delay,
  but pray to the Lord, and he will heal you.
Give up your faults and direct your hands rightly,
  and cleanse your heart from all sin. . . .
Then give the physician his place, for the Lord created
  him;
  do not let him leave you, for you need him.
There may come a time when recovery lies in the hands
  of the physicians,
  for they too pray to the Lord
that he grant them success in diagnosis
  and in healing, for the sake of preserving life.
(Ecclus 38:1-4, 9-14 NRSV)

Then comes the statement with which we started—"He who sins against his Maker, will be defiant toward the physician." He will thus show himself a fool, not only in the directly spiritual sense of not reckoning with the reality and claims of God (which is the mark of the fool throughout the canonical Wisdom literature), but also in the everyday sense of undervaluing something good and beneficial that God has provided for him, namely the skills and ministrations of the professional healer. Ecclesiasticus is not part of the canon of Scripture that Protestants acknowledge, but Anglican Article Six of the Thirty-nine speaks of it as one of the books "the Church doth read for example of life and instruction of manners," and this very positive view of medicine and the medical profession is one that Christians should not hesitate to accept. So I begin this address by inviting you to join with me in celebrating the God-given privilege and responsibility, the vital need and the noble task, of the professional medical work that you do.

Consider, now, your agenda for the next three days. The Conference theme is "Christian Character, Virtue, and Bioethics." The three days will be devoted to exploring successively the virtues of faith, hope, and love in medical practice. The aim will be to form a conceptual model of Christian and medical excellence combining in the life of the present-day practitioner in this part of the world. If the Conference theme had been announced as "The Virtuous Physician" it would have sounded quaint, old-fashioned, and not quite serious, for in the cynical English-speaking world of today "virtue" and "virtuous" in application to human beings are not far from being terms of mockery; but in strict dictionary terms—connotation terms, if you prefer the logician's lingo—these words, which speak of moral purpose and moral excellence in doing whatever it is that you do, are the words best expressing the ideal at which your agenda aims. And you have invited me, as a theologian, to kick-start you—which is what, as I understand it, keynote addresses as such are meant to do. It is a great privilege, but a daunting one. What can I bring to help you in your endeavours?

A theologian's stock-in-trade is theology, so I shall bring you theology—and I shall bring it to you in a specific way. C. S. Lewis, as I expect you know, wrote many articles by request for newspapers and magazines on a wide variety of themes; when asked on one occasion where he got his ideas of what to say on these topics, he replied that he asked himself what his grandmother (a voluble, scatterbrained Irish clergyman's wife) would have said, and then proceeded in his own style to say the same. Probably he was only half serious when he said that; but I am a good deal more than half serious when I tell you that I am following a comparable course. It was my privilege at one time to be close to the late David Martyn Lloyd-Jones, who at the age of twenty-seven gave up his job as personal assistant to Lord Horder, the then royal physician, and turned his back on his scintillating prospects as a consultant with an almost magical flair for diagnosis, in order to become a preacher and a pastor, in other words an evangelist and physician of souls, or rather, as he himself saw and said it, a healer of the whole person, whose treatment began with diagnosing and prescribing for the real root of human problems, namely sin. Lloyd-Jones was both the greatest preacher and teacher and the greatest man that I have known, and I imagine (for there is no way I can measure this) that there is more of him under my skin than there is of anyone else when it comes to defining and transmitting Christianity. I have asked myself, in light of things I heard him say and transcriptions of addresses that he gave over the years specifically to medical personnel,[1] what he would be telling you were he giving this address today, and I will not deny that what I say to you now will to some extent reflect my reflections on that point.

Furthermore, a theologian in my view is, or should be, a sort of pastor, certainly to the church at large and perhaps to individuals too. His responsibility under God is not primarily to his professional peers but to the church, just as a physician's primary responsibility is not to the professional guild but to his patients. Through his public debates and utterances, therefore, he must care for the Lord's sheep with proper shepherdly responsibility, guiding them away from places of danger and leading them to good pasture. That is how I see my own role, such as it is, in the kingdom of God. In this I consciously follow in the footsteps of the great Reformers, Luther and Calvin, who were pastors of congregations before they were anything else; and I follow in the footsteps also of the noble army of late sixteenth- and seventeenth-century Puritan clergymen—Anglican, Presbyterian, Congregational, and Baptist—who first coined and claimed the description of the pastor as a physician of the soul. They as a body were gifted theologians whose ministry was one of teaching the faith of the Reformation in an experiential Augustinian frame, and of leading people to conversion, holiness, assurance, love of God and neighbour, and community in the family and the church; and they fulfilled the applicatory dimension of their ministry, both from the pulpit and in what we would call personal pastoral direction, by means of a biblically formed technique of diagnosis and prescription that in my view is still way out in front of anything that is on public offer in the Protestant churches today.

I speak to you, therefore, as one who has come to resonate at a deep level with the medical way of working out what is best for those whom one seeks to serve in Christ. Perhaps this will become apparent as we go along; if so, I hope you will not take it amiss.

Faith

"Faith" is the first word in the title to which I have been asked to speak, and it is entirely appropriate that we should start our explorations here. For it is faith that gives us our Christian identity, that of being *believers*, and it is faith that gives us our basic attitudes to God, to humankind, and to things—or perhaps I should say here, to all created realities that are not distinctively human, including all lesser and simpler forms of life, both animal and vegetable, plus all those entities that have no biology. To be more specific:

First, faith gives us our attitude to God, the Father, the Son, and the Holy Spirit, the Three-in-One whom we acknowledge as Creator and Sustainer, constantly active in providence and grace. This is the God whom we recognize to be in every way transcendent and majestic; yet whom we trust and love and adore, because "his name to us is love," and he has stooped in love to make friends with us, and to assure us that he values our company now and for eternity. This is awesome, if anything ever was, yet by faith we know it to be true, and rejoice accordingly.

Second, faith gives us our attitude to ourselves, weak, silly, and sinful as we are. By faith we know ourselves as redeemed and regenerate sinners, called now to worship and serve the God who has saved us, is saving us, and will save us. In all that we do we are to honour him and seek to advance his praise and glory, knowing that as we do so we shall find within ourselves a sense of fulfilment and delight that is not attainable any other way. Living thus, our contentment grows, and our Christlikeness also.

Third, faith gives us our attitude to other people. In general, we are to see everyone with whom we have any contact at all as our neighbour, to be respected, loved, helped, and served according to what need he or she has and what power we have to assist. Then within this frame we are to give priority to fulfilling our obligations to family members and to fellow-believers and to any to whom we have committed ourselves by the bonds of explicit promises, or to whom we are bound by our or their position in society. We shall return to this shortly, when we reflect on the physician's covenantal commitment to his or her patients to seek the best for them.

Fourth, faith gives us our attitude to what was once called the created order and is nowadays called the environment. By faith we learn that God made our race stewards and managers of the environment, to develop and use it according to his scheme of values in our culture-building, which includes, of course, health care and all the technology and technique that we devise for that purpose. All-important for faith is the preservation of the God-given scale of values as a permanent frame for technical and experimental developments. The sanctity of life, the worth of the individual person, and the maximizing of well-being, which includes health, as an expression of neighbour-love, are three basic values to which faith holds, and must hold, tenaciously.

What, then, is faith in itself? Though often reduced, even in church circles, to orthodoxy without relational commitment, or else to optimism without cognitive warrant, faith is in fact a whole-souled intellectual and volitional response to a revelation of God that calls for a totally new mind-set, relationship, and way of life. Here is how the Westminster Confession states the matter, in its chapter fourteen titled "Of Saving Faith":

> The grace of faith, whereby the elect are enabled to believe to the saving of their souls, is the work of the Spirit of Christ in their hearts, and is ordinarily wrought by the ministry of the Word, by which also, and by the administration of the sacraments, and prayer, it is increased and strengthened.
>
> By this faith, a Christian believeth to be true whatsoever is revealed in the Word, for the authority of God himself speaking therein, and acteth differently upon that which each particular passage containeth; yielding obedience to the commands, trembling at the threatenings, and embracing the promises of God for this life, and that which is to come. But the principal acts of saving faith are accepting, receiving, and resting upon Christ alone for justification, sanctification, and eternal life, by virtue of the covenant of grace.

Faith, in other words, is knowledge plus responsive action. It is formed by the impact of its object through the agency of the Holy Spirit. Its overall object, speaking broadly and inclusively, is everything that the canonical Scriptures communicate as from God. Its focal object, speaking now with evangelical precision, is twofold: it is the Lord Jesus Christ, the incarnate Son of God, in the fullness of his mediatorial ministry and it is the gracious promises of a gracious

heavenly Father based on Christ's work of redemption and recon-
ciliation on the cross. Faith is the ear and eye of the soul perceiving
the Christ of the Scriptures, the arms of the soul embracing him as
the living Saviour and Lord, and the feet of the soul following him
as he summons us to do. Older theologians analyzed saving faith as
notitia (knowledge about Jesus Christ), *assensus* (acknowledgement
that this Christ is for real, and this gospel is true and good), and
fiducia (trust in Christ, and confidence that one is accepted through
him, in him, and by him)—and this is as true and full an analysis as
one can find anywhere.

Faith, then, makes the Christian—indeed, defines the Christian;
and the first requirement for fulfilling the role of a Christian physician is actually to be a Christian, one who has received and now follows Jesus Christ, seeking to practise love of God and love of neighbour according to Christ's teaching and example. Neighbour-love for
the glory of God will therefore be the category into which Christian
physicians will see their professional work fitting, and this will determine their spirit and attitude in tackling it. Which brings us to
the second of the topics on which I was asked to address you,
namely *covenant*, and the sense in which the physician-patient relationship should be regarded as *covenantal*.

Covenant

Covenant is the generic biblical word for any sort of bonded and
bonding relationship that carries obligations and expectations on
both sides. Scripture knows of covenants between husband and wife,
between friend and friend, between conqueror and conquered, and
between king and subjects. Also, and from one standpoint primarily,
in the Bible's account of God's saving activity his redemptive commitment to his people is regularly described as his covenant with
them; so we read of the *old* covenant established at Sinai, and of the
new covenant inaugurated by Jesus' blood-shedding; and in prophecy
and promise we repeatedly encounter what we can call the *slogan* of
God's covenant in both its old and its new forms—"I will be your
God; you shall be my people." Encountering this promise, we are
meant to understand that the commitment expressed by the pronoun in the phrase "*your* God" is a guarantee of privilege, protection, and endless enrichment to the redeemed, up to the limit of

God's resourcefulness in gracious giving; and we are also to understand that the obligation expressed by the pronoun in the phrase "my people" is to serve God and seek his praise in everything that we do, both in our direct worship and in our treatment of each other; and the third thing we must understand is that this obligation rests equally on every member of the group to which the promise is made—old Israel, that is, the genealogical seed of Abraham, in the days before Christ, and new Israel, the community of Christian believers who are the spiritual seed of Abraham, in the era that Christ's redemptive ministry began.

The phrases "old covenant" and "new covenant" for the two successive forms of God's conveyance of saving mercy to mankind, and the concept of "covenant theology" as a name for the systematic spelling out of these redemptive arrangements, are no doubt familiar to us all; but most of us would probably have to admit that our thinking about the covenantal dimensions of life stops there. However, Karl Barth, that most powerful of twentieth-century theologians, based his ethical thinking on the premise that all human life as such, under God and before his face, is covenantal, in the sense that as the Creator's blessing has already been received in the very fact that we are alive at all, so obligations to God and to our fellow human beings are, so to speak, built into our existence and must be consciously recognized and acknowledged as creational facts. The ethicist Paul Ramsey followed Barth in this, and I should like to quote his very clear account of the principle in the preface to his landmark exploration of medical ethics, titled *The Patient as Person.* Here, then, is Ramsey's statement.

> At crucial points in the analysis of medical ethics, I shall not be embarrassed to use as an interpretative principle the Biblical norm of *fidelity to covenant,* with the meaning it gives to *righteousness* between man and man. . . . I hold with Karl Barth that covenant-fidelity is the inner meaning and purpose of our creation as human beings, while the whole of creation is the external basis and condition of the possibility of covenant. This means that the conscious acceptance of covenant responsibilities is the inner meaning of even the "natural" or systemic relations into which we are born, and of the

institutional relations or roles we enter by choice, while this fabric [he means, everything around us, our environment, circumstances, and milieu] provides the external framework for human fulfillment in explicit covenants among men. The practice of medicine is one such covenant. *Justice, fairness, righteousness, faithfulness, the canons of loyalty,* the *sanctity* of human life, *hesed* [Hebrew word for loving-kindness or steadfast love] *agape* or *charity* are some of the names given to the moral quality of attitude and action owed to all men by any man who steps into a covenant with another man— by any man who . . . explicitly acknowledges that we [he means, we who make up the human race] are a covenant people on a common pilgrimage.

Ramsey then states his agenda.

The chief aim of the chapters to follow is, then, simply to explore the meaning of *care*, to find the actions and abstentions that come from adherence to *covenant*, to ask the meaning of the *sanctity* of life, to articulate the requirements of steadfast *faithfulness* to a fellow man.[2]

Exactly! This is the track on which medical ethics must ever travel, in this conference as in all other times and places. Surely the Barth-Ramsey anchoring of the concept of covenant in the created order, which in effect exhibits neighbour-love as natural law, and turns into genuine theology the Kantian axiom that a human being must never be treated merely as a means, but always as an end, is a line of thought that we should accept and build on for ourselves as we seek to pick our way through the thickets of the doctor-patient relationship.

There has been some discussion as to whether *covenant* or *contract* is the term that best expresses the appropriate ideal for this relationship in today's Western world. Some might wonder whether there is any deep difference of meaning between these words, and for some moderns there may not be, but for the Christian who accepts our reasoning thus far, covenant and contract are not the same thing at all. A contract is seen as a negotiated arrangement between humans in which mutual liability is limited by agreement, while a covenant is seen in terms of the line of thought just set out, as a divinely imposed relational bond, rooted in the reality first of creation and then of redemption; and in a covenant liability is limited only by the known need of the other party and the possibilities of service that the actual situation and role-relationship of the parties allow. Covenant, we might say, is from above, contract from below, and Christians will not use the first of these terms as a synonym for the second, but will reserve it for the expressing of this higher meaning.

Let us now look more closely at the arguing that goes on here. In favour of the contract idea it is maintained that:

1. the category of contract eliminates *authoritarianism* from the physician-patient relationship, since it inhibits the physician from behaving like a parent, priest, or mystagogue who has on his hands an immature and unintelligent child, and instead displays the relationship as one of free voluntary agreement between adults, in which full exchange and discussion of relevant information at each stage of the diagnosis and treatment is mandated;

2. the category of contract eliminates *exploitation* and *injustice* from the relationship, by providing recourse under the law for the patient to make the physician accountable under the contract for the quality of service rendered;

3. the category of contract eliminates *condescension* from the relationship, by moving it away from any supposed basis in social superiority or inferiority. As William May phrases it, "a contract does not rely on the pose of philanthropy or condescend as 'charity.' It presupposes frankly that self-interest governs people. When the two parties enter into a contract, they do so because each cuts a deal that serves his or her own advantage."[3] The contractual focusing of self-interest on both sides is held to bring realism into the understanding of what goes on when a physician is professionally consulted.

There is obvious substance for the correcting and avoiding of abuses in each of these three arguments, and I have nothing to say against them. The only point I wish to make is that for the Christian physician the contractual understanding of the relationship with the patient, along with all other aspects of the relationship—didactic, technical, instructional, and whatever else—must be set within a covenantal frame, in which the physician's obligation to render the best service he or she can in matters concerning the life, death, health, and well-being of one who is God's image bearer is primary. In other words, medical service as a social reality must be understood and undertaken as, quite precisely, neighbour-love. Contract within covenant must be the concept that guides; a contract intended for the fulfilling under God of covenant obligations to one's neighbour should be the Christian physician's constant view of the bond that operates in his or her professional commitments to each patient. To think through one's professional life and work in these terms may mean some swimming against the intellectual stream that flows here and there within the guild—Christian teachers in the public school system have similar problems—but it is a necessary discipline if one's professionalism is to be in truth service of God.

The Physician at Work

What guidelines, then, does Christian theology offer for hands-on medical practice? Speaking from the touchlines as I do (for I am only a theologian, after all), I see neighbour-love, both as a divine command and as a created instinct distorted by sin but now redemptively restored in each Christian's makeup, requiring from physicians fulfillment of the duty of covenantal care towards each patient—care in which personal well-being in both body and soul is the ultimate end in view. While medical care and pastoral evangelism are not the same thing, it is apparent that at this point of goal-setting the concerns of the Christian physician and the Christian pastor converge, in such a way that co-operation between them becomes natural and frequently necessary. The most difficult part of medical practice, as everyone knows, is doing the best you can for patients in less than ideal situations, where therapeutic trade-offs have to be made and the doing of most good, in the sense of relieving pain and maximizing ability to function humanly involves, by the inexorable law of double effect, that you do incidentally some harm. I do not wonder at the distress medical personnel sometimes undergo when faced by the need to make such decisions, as in relation to wasting and terminal conditions they often have to; I only wonder whether Christian medical personnel, at least, gain all the help they might in such cases from consulting with pastors and acquainting themselves with the long legacy of Christian thought on therapeutic themes.

But be that as it may, the twin qualities of *integrity* and *fidelity* in dealing with patients are most obviously required of Christian physicians, as belonging to both the ethical demands and the personal spirituality of their work. This twofold demand can be well anchored, and thereby focused, in the New Testament idea of the Christian life as "doing the truth" (Jn 3:21, cf. 1 Jn 1:6): that is, obeying God's truth, expressing it, and embodying it in its relation to the realities of life; "truthing it in love" as many during the past century have translated a pregnant participle in Ephesians 4:15.[4] On this, and what it involves, I would like to quote some magisterial paragraphs from William May, whose statement as it seems to me could hardly be bettered. In his handbook on medical ethics, *The Physician's Covenant*, from which I have quoted already, he is explaining how the covenantal concept that we have been reviewing calls for and leads to "a pervasive fidelity that informs the performance of all duties," and he labours to nail this fidelity down in specifics, lest it "lapse into an indeterminate earnestness." (O wise man!—I speak as a pastor: how much fuzzy-headed, indeterminate earnestness there is around! and how much need we have across the Christian board for clear and hard heads to accompany warm hearts!) On the Christian physician's fidelity in communicating truth about the patient's condition within the truth of the covenantal bond between them, now, May writes as follows:

> The professional quandary of truth-telling nicely demonstrates the difference a covenantal ethic can make in practice. Moralists usually reduce the quandary of telling the truth to the question of whether to tell the truth. Consequentialists seek to answer the question by calculating the goods and harms produced by the truth, evasion, or lying. They prize the virtue of benevolence. Duty-oriented moralists tend to argue for the truth irrespective of consequences. A lie wrongs the patient even when it does no harm. Managing the patient, even for benevolent reasons, subverts the patient's dignity. Only the truth respects the patient as a rational creature. Such moralists thus prize foremost here the virtue of honesty.
>
> The virtue of covenantal fidelity expands the question

of truth-telling in the moral life. Truth becomes a question not only of telling the truth but of being-true. . . .

J. I. [sic: should be L.] Austin once drew the distinction, now famous, between two kinds of utterances: descriptive and performative. In ordinary descriptive sentences, one points to or characterizes a given item in the world. (It is raining, The tumor is malignant.) In performative utterances, however, one alters the world by introducing an ingredient that would not be there apart from the utterance. Promises make such performative declarations. (I, John, take thee, Mary. We will defend your country in case of attack. I will not abandon you.) To make a promise alters the world of the person to whom one extends the promise. Conversely, defecting from a promise can be world shattering. . . .

The notion of performative speech expands the question of truth-telling in professional life. Physicians and nurses face the moral question not simply of telling the truth, but of being true to their word. Conversely, the total situation for a patient includes not only the disease one has but also whether others desert or stand by a person in this extremity. The fidelity of others will not eliminate the disease, but it affects mightily the human context in which the disease runs its course. The doctor offers a patient not simply proficiency and diagnostic accuracy but also fidelity.

Thus the virtue of fidelity begins to affect the resolution of the dilemma itself. Perhaps more patients and clients could accept the descriptive truth if they experienced the performative truth. The anxieties of patients in terminal illness compound because they fear that professionals will abandon them . . . a cautiously wise medieval physician once advised his colleagues: "Promise only fidelity!"[5]

This admirable indication of how a physician's Christian faith will express itself in a covenantal fidelity to the patient that can perfectly be described as "truthing it in love" leaves me with nothing more to say; so now I close. In a secular society, Christian physicians are precious people, and it is important that they not lose their edge. Covenantal professionalism will keep one's edge keen. To commend it, as I have been doing, is a privilege and a joy. By it humans are blessed, and God is glorified: may there then be more of it as the years go by. This is the way that we must go, for it is truly the path of faith and love, whereby the physician serves and follows our Lord and Saviour Jesus Christ.

Notes

1 D. Martyn Lloyd-Jones, *Healing and the Scriptures* (Nashville, Tenn.: Oliver-Nelson, 1988).

2 Paul Ramsey, *The Patient as Person* (New Haven, Conn.: Yale University Press, 1975), xii–xiii.

3 William F. May, *The Physician's Covenant: Images of the Healer in Medical Ethics* (Philadelphia: Westminster Press, 1983), 117.

4 The participle signifies "not only speaking truth but living and acting it as well." F. F. Bruce, *The Epistle to the Ephesians* (London: Pickering and Inglis, 1961), 88. Renderings offered by commentators include "dealing truly," "living the truth," "adhering to the truth," "practising sincerity," "practising integrity," "maintaining, living, and doing the truth," "following the truth."

5 May, 142–43.

Jan Hux

Toward a Christian Ethic of Health Care Financing and Physician Reimbursement

I n *The Doctor's Dilemma*, George Bernard Shaw contended that it was absurd to give the surgeon a pecuniary interest in cutting off a patient's leg. Had he been writing in the era of managed care, he might have just as strongly asserted that it was absurd to give the physician a pecuniary interest in cutting off a patient's access to health services. Certainly the financing and reimbursement of health services is a field rife with perverse incentives and across industrialized countries over the past four decades policies designed to eliminate one particular set of these incentives, have merely opened the door for a different set of counterproductive practices. The blueprint for a health system which will provide adequate but not excessive health services on an equitably distributed basis and within a reasonably constrained budget probably does not exist—at least it will not be found in this essay. What I seek to do in this paper is to describe in broad terms some of the payment schemes that are currently in use, describe the incentives inherent in them and their implications for access to care. Finally, I will attempt to identify some of the ethical issues raised by these policies—points of tension for Christians seeking to "act justly and to love mercy and to walk humbly with [our] God" (Mic 6:8 NIV).

The Function of Health Insurance
Almost every industrialized nation relies on some form of health insurance as a means to finance health care. There are exceptions such as Singapore which has a mandatory employee health savings

plan from which individuals purchase health services when they require them. However, the purchasing of medical services for infrequent and often unpredictable illnesses at costs that are potentially overwhelming lends itself extremely well to a program of insurance as a way to reduce individual risk.

Insurance can be thought of as a means of transferring wealth, primarily a transfer to individuals who suffer loss as the result of an unpredictable event, from those who were similarly at risk but did not sustain a loss. Thus, health insurance transfers wealth from the well to the sick, much as fire insurance transfers wealth from those whose houses are intact to one whose house has burned down. However, health insurance can be extended to facilitate two types of transfers not usually seen in other fields of insurance: transfers from low-risk individuals to high-risk individuals and from the rich to the poor. The former might be accomplished, for instance, by offering insurance to the elderly or the chronically ill at the same premium as young healthy individuals even though it is probable that they will use far more services—this, in contrast to auto insurance where high-risk drivers face higher premiums. The latter, transfers from rich to poor, may be achieved by financing health insurance out of tax revenues (assuming a progressive taxation scheme).

What do these "transfers of wealth" mean in practical terms? Transfers from well to sick mean that when a young woman with appendicitis arrives at the hospital she will have access to care without having to pay out-of-pocket. The event was unpredictable so her insurer could not have charged her a higher premium in anticipation of the loss. Her fellow policy holders are willing to pay for her care and don't require her to be financially penalized because each realizes that "it could have been me."

But what happens to this young woman's brother when he gets diabetes? Under a traditional private insurance scheme, risks are pooled among individuals who have a similar probability of an event. The young man would join a pool of higher risk individuals for whom an actuarially fair premium is considerably higher than that paid by his healthy sister. We may wonder whether it is right that he should pay more simply because he is sick—after all, the purpose of insurance was to protect him from illness related costs. At the same time, he will clearly use more services in the coming years and should he not pay for what he uses? The analogy to experience-rated automobile insurance is clear. Premiums are higher for teen-aged male drivers as a means of recovering costs they will incur but also as an attempt to reduce utilization.

Private Insurance

Nations have varied in the way in which insurance for medical services and hospitalization is provided, but I will simplify the range of options to three: private insurance, public insurance, and a combination of the two. The first of these, private insurance purchased by individuals or groups in a competitive market, has been the predominant model of health insurance in the United States. It provides a wide choice of plans with differing levels of coverage and co-payment schemes at a corresponding range of prices. Individuals obtain the level of coverage they are willing to pay for and are not forced to pay for coverage which they decide they will not need. One of the strongest criticisms of such a system is that individuals with chronic illness, identifiable risk factors, or even solo (as opposed to group) purchaser status usually face premiums which are prohibitively expensive.[1] Once the large pool of relatively young, healthy workers has been covered in employee group plans, premiums for others may rise to such an extent that low- and moderate-risk individuals conclude that insurance is not worth what it will cost them, and leave the market. Then, with only very high-risk individuals left in the pool, premiums rise even higher to cover the increased expected losses and even more buyers are forced out of the market—as it has been described, the "bad money drives out the good." Thus, under competitive private insurance schemes, the sick and elderly who are most likely to require health care have the greatest difficulty obtaining it.

Not only do commercial insurers set premiums which make it difficult for the chronically ill to obtain coverage, those who have coverage often face substantial co-payments and deductibles. These co-payments are intended to serve as a financial barrier and to thereby reduce utilization. If these measures selectively reduced frivolous use of health services, they would be an effective means to lower costs without impairing health outcomes. However this is not what has been observed. In the RAND health insurance experiment, utilization of services was most significantly reduced in patients in the lowest income segment of the population; and, as a result, these individuals had poorer outcomes on several health measures.[2] Other studies have found that financial barriers are as likely to reduce necessary care as frivolous or discretionary care.[3] For instance, when New Hampshire reduced the level of drug benefit coverage under Medicaid, it was observed that a substantial proportion of persons who had previously been receiving insulin and diuretics stopped obtaining these medications.[4] It seems unlikely that these drugs were being used frivolously prior to the policy change (particularly insulin) or that the policy change cured the patients of their diabetes or heart failure! Some patients were admitted to hospitals and long term care facilities because of a decline in health status, and even though the drug payment policy was later reversed, most of these patients never returned to independent living arrangements.[5]

It appears then, that under private insurance schemes, health care will be less accessible to the poor and the sick. One might observe that ski trips to Whistler, B.C., are also less accessible to the poor and sick but that such inequality is not necessarily problematic or in need of redress. Most of us however, see health care as different from a ski trip or other consumer commodities. Because of the implicit connection between the provision of health care and life and health which are themselves seen as rights, access to essential health services is usually, by extension, seen as a right. Most would argue that health care is different and that its distribution must therefore be treated differently.

To begin, we may object to a system of health care financing which reduces access for the poor and chronically ill, on strictly practical or economic grounds. A healthy work force may be seen as a worthwhile investment for a society much in the same way as our interest in an educated work force has motivated investment in public education. Purely selfish motives may prompt our desire to see that others get health care in the case of infectious diseases: for instance it is in my own best interest to see that my neighbour gets a full course of therapy for his tuberculosis infection. Some might argue that we may as well provide care to the indigent since, even in our increasingly secular society, a patient presenting *in extremis* at an emergency department who has neither insurance nor means to pay directly will not be denied care. (Economists refer to such an individual who foregoes insurance knowing he will not be denied charity care in the end as the "bleeding cheat.") If we choose to provide insurance to those who, because of elevated risk or low income, can not afford it, doing so through commercial providers will be more expensive than public insurance because of the propensity of private insurers to risk-select. Thus, subsidized private insurance may not be the most economically efficient means of providing coverage.[6]

Turning from economic arguments to ethics, the strong evidence that a purely private insurance program will reduce access to health services for both the poor and chronically ill, suggests that it violates the principle of justice in the allocation of health care. Such an interpretation presumes that the "health care" of which we are speaking consists of an effective use of medical services which would be expected to lead to improved health for the recipients, and that health care is not just another commodity which is to be rationed by price but, like access to justice, is expected to be available to all, regardless of ability to pay. An understanding that the value of life originates from the individual's creation in the image of God and not from the individual's socio-economic status or chronic health status implies that medical treatments to preserve that life should not be rationed on the basis of ability to pay or on external judgments of quality of life.

Finally, as Christians, we are especially called to care for the poor, the chronically ill ("the lame"), and the needy, not out of economic self-interest, nor merely in defence of the principles of justice, but as a practical expression of the gospel of grace. This may mean being an active advocate for methods of financing health care which do not discriminate against the poor and the sick. Where such methods fail, and patients face discriminatory barriers to care, it may mean going outside of the system to provide care. I should digress here briefly with a word about "charity" care. Certainly the medical profession has a long tradition of providing free care to those in real need who could not afford to pay. Care provided free of charge is a more tangible expression of charity or grace since it affects the physician's income directly (through the foregone earnings from caring for a paying patient) as opposed to care provided under public insurance where the physician bears only a small portion of the cost and then only very indirectly through the paying of tax. However, in a medical environment of increasing technological complexity, direct physician services comprise only a minor proportion of health care costs (in the order of 20%) such that a physician's willingness to forego his/her fee does little to remove the barriers to diagnostic, therapeutic, and hospital services that the patient may need. Charity care may still be feasible in a primary care setting but even there it generally requires a mix of patients so that the "paying patients" subsidize the care of those who cannot pay (although the adequacy of this cross-subsidization cannot be guaranteed as prairie physicians in the 1930s, forced to join bread lines with their patients, learned).

Public Insurance

In contrast to private insurance, public insurance not only redistributes wealth from the well to the sick but also from low-risk to high-risk individuals and from the rich to the poor. With universal insurance by a single payer, the insurer is not able to risk-select and individuals who would be predicted to have a greater need for health services are not priced out of the market.

Although they theoretically provide barrier-free access to care, single-payer health insurance systems have come under criticism. The lack of a competitive stimulus or profit motive and the sheer size of the plans is thought to preclude managerial efficiency. Because such a system does not place financial barriers in front of patients, there is a strong incentive for overuse, particularly in settings (such as most in Canada) where first dollar coverage of costs is combined with fee-for-service reimbursement of physicians. Such a system eliminates the negative aspects of rationing care on the basis of ability to pay, however, it must substitute some other form of rationing.

The need for rationing is never pleasant to contemplate—we would like to think we can offer every potentially helpful intervention to everyone but this is not feasible on several grounds. In the first place, the menu of available and "potentially helpful" interventions continues to grow with each new entry seemingly more expensive than the last, yet health care budgets are at best static. For reasons alluded to above as well as many others, health care is not like other goods and services—the criteria for perfect competition in which market forces are expected to lead to the most economically efficient distribution of resources are not met either in the market for health insurance or in the market for health services. To look at it another way, we want health, but all that we can purchase is health care. Since no amount of health care will lead to perfect health, we will always want or demand more. A system in which health care is financed through private insurance controls that demand by placing financial barriers in front of patients in the form of co-payments, deductibles, and high premiums. In contrast, a publicly funded system in which patients receive first dollar coverage manages the tendency to over-demand by constraining the supply of health services. Some have described this as rationing by waiting list. It is interesting that in Canada–United States comparisons, the feature of the other system which seems most repugnant to arm-chair analysts on one side of the border is the very means by which utilization is controlled on the other side of the border. Canadians are appalled at the notion that some Americans have care withheld because they are unable to pay and similarly Americans are incredulous that we put up with a system in which patients may wait for a year to get hip replacements.

The problem with rationing by waiting, or more accurately by supply constraint, is that, compared to rationing by price, it is much harder to do, and harder still to do well. Rationing by ability to pay is easy—the provider sets the price and it is left up to the patients to determine what services they are or are not willing to pay for. In contrast, rationing by queue requires that at the policy level decisions be made regarding which services will be made available, in what quantity, and to which patients. At the clinical level, the provider must determine how to function as patient advocate, seeking the best treatments within the available resources.

The weaknesses of such a basis for rationing are clear—patients may not be appropriately queued and may suffer excess morbidity and even mortality because of delayed access to care;[7] physicians may feel constrained in their capacity to provide optimal care and may feel forced into an uncomfortable role as gatekeeper. Physicians are quick to point out examples of clinical insensitivity on the part of policy makers and administrators as they make resource allocation decisions. Perhaps more troublesome is that in many cases, there is insufficient hard evidence about which treatments have the potential to benefit which patients.[8] As a result, decisions are not made at the policy level and rationing is forced down into the clinical realm. For instance in the case of cholesterol lowering in primary prevention, there is marked disagreement among expert panels, and in Ontario no clear policy has been articulated. Hence a primary care provider whose patient asks her about checking his cholesterol level may face a conflict between her desire to provide her patient with any intervention which may be of benefit and her need to respond to global pressures to decrease utilization. She knows that the potential benefit is likely to be very small if any, yet she cannot tell her patient that his small potential gain "isn't worth spending the money on."

The benefits of this means of rationing, apart from its capacity to reduce expenditures, are not as apparent; however it can be instructive to consider an alternative environment—one where supply is not constrained and in fact excess supply is provided in order to eliminate queuing. In a setting of excess supply, as the rate of a procedure increases, it will tend to be applied to patients for whom the benefits are progressively smaller and smaller,[9] and eventually to patients for whom the risks exceed the benefits. A hypothetical comparison of coronary artery bypass surgery in Ontario[10] and one of the western states[11] serves to illustrate the issues. In Ontario, rates of bypass surgery are about 750 cases per million adults, in the United States they range from 1,200 to 2,000 per million. The queue in Ontario is arranged such that the most urgent cases are done promptly but 25% of patients wait more than seven weeks for surgery, with an overall death rate of 0.4% on the queue. In America there is excess supply so that cases are done promptly, however in the face of this excess capacity, surgery is performed on some patients for whom it is inappropriate (risks clearly exceed the benefits), with an inappropriateness rate of 14% found in the state which was studied. Recall that bypass surgery is a major cardiac procedure with a mortality rate of about 2%. Considering the hypothetical provision of bypass surgery for a population of one million adults, in Ontario, 750 cases would be done and three persons would die while awaiting surgery; in the western state, 1,500 cases might be done with no deaths from delay but there would be 210 cases in which the procedure was clearly inappropriate, and in four of these cases the patient would die from surgery which should not have been undertaken in the first place. In another 30% of cases the surgery, though not inappropriate, was not deemed clearly necessary, representing an additional 450 cases and nine additional perioperative deaths. While the numbers in this example may be disputed, the message is clear that in a supply-constrained environment patients may suffer from delayed or denied access to beneficial procedures, however in a system without supply constraints, patients will suffer the adverse effects of procedures which they did not require. Neither system is free of problems. The burden imposed by queuing will depend in part on how well the queue is managed, and it would be misleading to suggest that all queues are functioning as efficiently as that for bypass surgery in Ontario. For instance, in the case of total joint replacement (hip or knee repairs), unacceptably long queues persist in most areas of Ontario and only weak correlation is found between symptom severity and promptness of care.[12]

In an environment then, where health care is financed though publicly funded insurance, financial barriers to accessing care seen in the private insurance model are largely removed. All can freely access the system but the system cannot afford to provide all things to all people. So the ethical problems associated with public insurance arise not in access to care, but from the means used to control utilization and their impact on the nature of the care to which patients have access. Since patients do not directly bear the cost of their care and since physicians profit from delivering more care, there is an incentive to overuse services. This tendency to overuse is managed by restricting the availability of services (supply side constraints). The limited resources are allocated, at least in the ideal, on the basis of need. So, for instance, in a well-managed bypass surgery queue, a patient with severe disease (left mainstem lesion) and unmanageable symptoms will receive surgery within a week while one with minimal disease will not receive it at all, with no reference to his ability to pay. Some patients will suffer adverse outcomes while waiting on the queue but others will be spared the burden of a high proportion of unnecessary or inappropriate care.

In this model, ethical concerns arise at several levels. I have indicated that the rationing decisions—what types of health services will be made available to what types of patients and in what quantity—should be made at the policy level rather than at the bedside. When these decisions are made, they must be made on the basis of evidence of medical benefit or lack thereof, or on the basis of lack of evidence. As an example of the former, mammography is available for screening purposes for women over the age of fifty but not for younger women, since screening has been shown to reduce breast cancer deaths in the older group but to offer no benefit in younger women. An example of a lack of evidence driving policy would be the decision not to make PSA available in screening for prostate cancer, since there is no evidence that screening prolongs life or reduces morbidity. Decisions must not be made on the basis of arbitrary or subjective assessments about the quality or value of the life to be preserved by the intervention. Thus it may be appropriate to deny complex surgery to a ninety-year old with heart failure because for her the risks of the procedure clearly outweigh the benefits, but not because she is a chair-bound nonagenarian whose quality of life the provider deems to be unacceptable.

While the notion of rationing at the policy level is appealing on an ethical front since it frees the physician to act as a patient advocate rather than a health system advocate and on a scientific front because it facilitates patterns of care based on research outcomes, in practice it is often difficult if not impossible to achieve. In the first instance, as noted above, very often there is not sufficient evidence available on which to base a uniform policy. Where evidence does exist, it often reveals that the intervention yields a range of benefits for a range of patients and does not support a simple decision to either implement or prohibit the intervention. Policy initiatives may be tools which are too blunt to respond appropriately to the widely varying condition of patients even within a single diagnostic group. Policy-makers and expert panels may help to delineate the evidence in the form of a guideline, but the application to an individual patient will still need to occur at the bedside within the realm of the art of medicine.

Because rationing at the policy level is often impractical, there will be a tendency for the decisions to be pushed down into the clinical realm where they threaten the role of the physician as a "perfect agent" for the patient. The physician in an agency relationship assumes responsibility for directing the health care utilization of the patient, not as a profit-maximizing provider or as guardian of the provincial purse, but as an agent trying to choose what the patient would have chosen, had she been as well-informed as the professional.[13] Consider a physician who believes that treatment A offers the possibility of a slight clinical advantage over treatment B but is aware that it comes at a thirty-fold greater price. He may be operating under an institutional policy which requires him to use A (for instance a hospital radiology department which has refused to fund non-ionic contrast medium except for patients with a documented adverse reaction). He may be in an environment where the cost differential is borne by the patient (for instance graduated co-payment or reference pricing) and where he and the patient can assess together whether the chance of a small clinical benefit is worth it for that patient. Or he may simply be left with a conflict between the pressure to contain costs and to provide the best care for his patient.

One final issue that relates to how we should function as ethical physicians in a supply-constrained environment is the importance of eliminating unnecessary care. In situations where an expensive treatment offers a small marginal therapeutic advantage we experience conflict between our role as the patient's agent and the system's gatekeeper, however in situations where the expensive treatment or test offers no advantage we need to act responsibly by not using it. This is not to say that physicians are solely responsible for inappropriate expenditures in the health care system. We may not be able to control the patient who books an office appointment for what turns out to have been a frivolous reason, nor can we control the component of hospitalization costs that is created by administrative hypertrophy, but there are costs that we can control. Unnecessarily expensive drugs are widely used both because the aggressive marketing of these agents is effective and because prescribers are not aware of the price differentials involved. In Ontario in 1992, the drug benefit program covering seniors spent $12.9 million on two antibiotics, neither of which is considered first-line therapy for the outpatient management of infections commonly seen in the elderly but whose price exceeds that of some first-line agents by twenty-fold. These two drugs accounted for 55% of the antibiotic expenditures yet in the majority of cases their use would be difficult to justify. More conservative prescribing could have saved in the order of $10 million—that is $1,000 for every primary care physician in the province. In 1993, more than two million thyroid function tests were performed in Ontario—one for every five residents at a cost of more than $50 million. Given the prevalence of thyroid disease in the community, it is difficult to imagine that this level of testing is necessary. We need to be good stewards of the resources that are available. If we do not wish to be restricted in our ability to provide beneficial interventions to our patients then we need to be careful not to waste resources on interventions that will not benefit them. End of life care is another area identified as consuming unnecessary resources. In a recent survey of Canadian Intensive Care Unit directors, the most common cause of providing futile care identified by physicians was their own inability to come to terms with death and with their failure to provide a cure.[14] As Christian physicians we have a tremendous amount to contribute in defining appropriate end of life care, not to mention in responding to the spiritual needs of our colleagues for whom death is such a fearsome spectre.

To summarize, publicly funded care guarantees access independent of patients' ability to pay or pre-existing illness, but the system to which patients gain access has a restricted menu of choices with waiting lists for specialty services and may create a conflict for physicians between their responsibility to a patient and their responsibility to patients (i.e., the whole population of health service users).

Combined Public and Private Insurance

A third scheme for financing health care would be through a combination of public and private plans—not a patchwork as seen in the United States where some have public insurance (Medicare, Medicaid) while others operate in a quite independent realm of private insurance, but rather a universal public system covering all essential services beyond which it is permissible to purchase supplemental private insurance. Advocates of such a system suggest that it combines the best of both worlds—free access for those who could not afford care in a fully privatized system, yet efficient and timely delivery of expensive, high tech services for those able and willing to pay. Cynics would demur that it merely provides the worst of both worlds —overutilization in the high-capacity private arm and decreased efficiency in the public arm.

Most of the problems with a system of mixed public and private insurance are apparent from the preceding discussion of the weaknesses in the individual components, but there are some issues which are unique to a blended system. The first of these is the assumption that it is possible to define a body of "essential" or "basic" services which should be fully covered in the public plan. The Oregon Medicaid experience suggests that the published cost-effectiveness literature is woefully inadequate for such a task and when Oregon planners attempted to use it, it provided such nonsense results as ranking jaw splints for TMJ dysfunction ahead of surgery for ruptured ectopic pregnancy. If we say that the only essential services are those which preserve life, we end up with another set of unacceptable conclusions such as the provision of expensive surgery (liver transplant, coronary bypass for left mainstem disease) but denial of palliative care (morphine for terminal cancer pain). If we revise our list to include any treatment which provides either life extension or symptom relief, then the issue becomes what additional services could be offered under supplemental private insurance. If such additional services would not make the private patients either feel better or live longer, it is not clear that it is to their benefit to receive them. Perhaps private insurance would serve simply to make the same services available but without the delays experienced in the public system. This rapid access would not be problematic for items such as diagnostic procedures where private patients could access an independent private facility. However for complex therapeutic interventions such as bypass surgery, where the care would be provided in competition with public patients, it could be argued that it would be unethical to allow private patients to "jump the queue" and displace public patients with much more severe disease for whom the procedure could be lifesaving.

Under a dual coverage system, patients who purchase supplemental insurance would be anticipated to access more care and experience fewer delays. However, as was illustrated in the case of the provision of bypass surgery in a setting of excess capacity, giving patients all of the health services they are willing to pay for (or buy insurance to cover), may not be serving their best interests. For other economic goods it is axiomatic that "more is better," but in the provision of health services, more is often *not* better and in fact more may be harmful. In a system where patients can purchase unlimited quantities of health care, it will be important to protect them from the ill-effects of over-use. This is not meant to imply that physicians are recommending procedures which they know to be inappropriate to their ill-informed and vulnerable patients, rather, that it is only natural that clinicians come to assume that the care they deliver is efficacious, that physicians do have a bias toward action ("when in doubt, cut it out") and that for a large proportion of the management decisions physicians routinely make, the scientific literature does not provide an unequivocal answer about a particular action's appropriateness or inappropriateness.

Finally, one of the dangers of a "two-tiered" system is that once the wealthy, vocal, and politically active members of society have left the public system in order to receive care on the private side, there will no longer be adequate pressure to maintain quality in the public system. As one health services researcher has put it, we need to keep the canaries inside the mine. Physicians providing care in the public component of a dual system will need to be particularly vigilant as patient advocates in attempting to ensure adequate service levels and quality.

Physician Reimbursement

The first half of this paper described means by which the health care system could be funded; the remainder examines how those funds should be used to reimburse physicians for their services. The reimbursement of hospital services, drugs, and diagnostic services will not be examined. As in the case of health insurance strategies, there are several broad categories of physician reimbursement plans.[15] These will be described, their incentives and impact on utilization patterns will be explored and ethical problems they raise will be identified.

Fee For Service

Under a fee-for-service (FFS) reimbursement plan, as the name implies, physicians are paid a specified sum for each service they deliver. Fees, under provincial plans in Canada, are established in a negotiated fee schedule that is applied province-wide. Individual physicians are not able to alter the fee they receive for a particular service, however they can control their income by altering the number or type of services provided. A FFS system presents a strong volume incentive to physicians, which makes it difficult for payers (the provincial health plans) to control expenditures. As a consequence, payers resort to a variety of measures to try to regain control of the cost of physicians' services. For instance, a hard cap may be applied to the budget for physicians services such that expenditures beyond that cap are recovered from physicians either by holdbacks or clawbacks.

A FFS system presents physicians with two incentives which can lead to undesirable outcomes. The first of these, as noted above, is the incentive to provide a high volume of services. Depending on the nature of the services, excess utilization may create a burden for patients and even lead to adverse outcomes. The relative valuation of services within the fee schedule also creates its own incentives which may lead to an inefficient allocation of health services. Since procedures are much more lucrative than counselling or patient education, the patient may get too little of the latter and too many of the former.

The second undesirable incentive in a FFS environment with a capped global budget is to pursue one's own interests at the expense of colleagues' interests. As a physician billing under such a plan, it is in my best interest to bill very large amounts and have all my colleagues bill modest amounts. This places me at a high starting income, but, since I'm the only one with a high income, the global cap will not be exceeded and I will not face a clawback. Unfortunately for me, the same incentives are acting on each of the other individual physicians billing under the plan. This is an example of the well described common-property resource phenomenon.[16] A familiar illustration will be the east coast fish stocks. It is in a single fisherman's best interest to fish as much as he pleases but have all the other fishermen stay within tight quotas so that the stocks aren't depleted. Each one's individual interest is in conflict with the collective interest. All users are penalized by the inappropriate and selfish actions of a few. It will be tempting in such an environment to say that because we know the clawback is coming and because everyone else is padding their billing, we need to do so too, so that we are not being disproportionately penalized. Living by the virtue of faith, however, does not leave room for such behaviour. We need to practise and to bill with full integrity, trusting to God to protect our interests as we walk in obedience to him.

Capitation

Under a capitation payment scheme, a physician receives a set sum for each patient enrolled in his or her practice. This eliminates the volume incentive inherent in the FFS system and provides more predictable charges to the payer. Since the physician doesn't experience pressure to "push the patients through" or perform procedures in order to generate revenue, there is greater opportunity to spend time with individual patients. There is also an incentive to provide quality care in that if an unhappy patient leaves the practice, the physician's income is reduced. The disadvantage of such a system is that while it removes the incentive for excess utilization, it may not promote a sufficient level. This has been partly addressed in the British primary care setting through the provision of FFS volume incentives for preventive services (i.e., base payment is on a capitation basis but a volume bonus is provided for immunizations and cervical cancer screening).

A second danger under capitation is a disincentive to care for patients with complex medical problems—if one is paid the same amount to care for a patient with AIDS, one with severe heart failure, or a healthy twenty year old, there is a strong incentive to take on the latter. This may be compensated for by applying a severity adjustment to the base capitation fee; however these adjustments can be complex to use while still inadequately precise. In the American HMO setting where many physicians are under capitation arrangements, they may also bear a financial risk associated with the cost of the tests and treatments they order for their patients, a further disincentive to providing an adequate quantity of care. Thus, a capitated system frees physicians from the high-volume treadmill of a straight FFS plan; at the same time, it places them in an environment where they will need to work to guard access for their patients, particularly for those whose health status requires a high quantity of care.

Salary

In a salaried environment, payment for all services delivered over a period of time is aggregated into one pre-specified lump sum. In general, while such an arrangement provides a predictable income, it has been presumed to be unacceptable to physicians because a full-time salaried position implies an employer. Payers may also value the predictability of charges that they will incur with salaried physicians but may have difficulty ensuring an adequate volume of services will be delivered in the absence of any volume incentive. (In managed care settings such as some American HMOs where physicians are salaried, the employer can ensure volume by booking large numbers of patient visits; however, this level of control is not feasible in settings where the connection between payer, provider, and insurer is not so direct.) Since a salaried arrangement fails to provide physicians with incentives to deliver either an adequate quantity of service (income not linked to volume) or high quality (income not jeopardized by patients leaving to get care elsewhere), it is unlikely to be widely adopted.

For each of the commonly used physician reimbursement schemes, physicians are placed in a position, with greater or lesser frequency, where they need to choose between self-interest (maximizing income or maximizing leisure time) and the patient's best interest (receiving adequate but not excessive care delivered in a compassionate manner). Those seeking to walk by faith should not require direct financial incentives to provide an appropriate quantity and quality of care. As Christian physicians we should work to achieve a just allocation of health services and our delivery of those services should reflect the grace of the gospel, the grace of him who said "freely you have received, freely give."

The Virtue of Faith

Finally I would like to take a step back and reconnect with the context for this paper—Christian ethics, and more specifically, the virtue of faith. The area of physician reimbursement will be a sensitive topic for a number of the doctors hearing or reading this paper. It is difficult not to be infected with the disillusionment, anger, and despair of our colleagues who feel betrayed by a health care system in which they have invested their lives. Those who trained in the 1970s do not have the health care system which they were promised—relative incomes have dropped from 5.6 times the national average in 1971 to just over 3 times a decade later, many feel that the physicians' role has shifted from the delivery of care to the rationing of care and on the patient side, the level of respect and esteem automatically accorded physicians has been substantially eroded over the past twenty-five years. The prognosis can look gloomy. Yet God has not been unfaithful to us and his promises to us remain unbroken. The Lord's hand is not shortened by the provincial ministry of health and his ability to meet our needs is not constrained by the national debt. Dependence on God's faithful provision for us rather than strident defence of our "right" to a particular income needs to be our starting point if we are to exercise the virtue of faith in this matter of physician reimbursement.

Some may argue that in seeking a health care system that justly delivers care to all patients, we are being pushed toward a system which fails to justly reimburse physicians. Some may point out that St. Paul teaches that the worker deserves his wage (1 Tim 5:18) (though Paul's context was the preaching of the gospel, not the delivery of health services). I would remind you that Paul also said "but if we have food and clothing, with these we shall be content" (1 Tim 6:6-8 RSV) and "I know how to be abased and how to abound, in any and all circumstances I have learned the secret of facing plenty and hunger, abundance and want" (Phil 4:12 RSV). If, in the context of the current medical funding "crisis," even a few physicians are forced to acknowledge their dependence on God and learn the secret of being content in all circumstances, then the crisis will in fact have been a blessing. If, in the context of intense financial pressure where it seems impossible to get ahead, some are forced to acknowledge that mammon is an intolerable master and turn afresh to single-hearted service to God, then those pressures will have been truly freeing.

As Christians we need to make our voice heard in the current wave of massive health care restructuring. However, we need to do that out of a certainty that it is God who provides for us, not the provincial ministry of health or the efforts of our own hands (Deut 8:17, 18). From that stance, we can argue not out of economic self interest but from a commitment to see health care allocated justly and delivered with mercy and compassion. May God give us grace to do so.

Notes

1 R. G. Evans, *Strained Mercy: The Economics of Canadian Health Care* (Toronto: Butterworths, 1984), ch. 2.

2 R. H. Brook et al., "Does Free Care Improve Adults' Health? Results from a Randomized Controlled Trial," *New England Journal of Medicine* 309 (1983): 1426-34.

3 M. F. Shapiro et al., "Out-of-Pocket Payments and Use of Care for Serious and Minor Symptoms. Results of a National Survey," *Archives of Internal Medicine* 149 (1989): 1645-48; B. Foxman, K. N. Lohr, and R. B. Valdez, "The Effect of Cost-Sharing on the Use of Antibiotics in Ambulatory Care: Results from a Population Based Randomized Controlled Trial," *Journal of Chronic Diseases* 40 (1987): 429-37; A. L. Siu et al., "Inappropriate Use of Hospitals in a Randomized Trial of Health Insurance Plans," *New England Journal of Medicine* 315 (1986): 1259-66.

4 S. B. Soumerai, D. Ross-Degrasy, and J. Avorn, "Payment Restrictions for Prescription Drugs Under Medicaid: Effects on Therapy, Cost and Equity," *New England Journal of Medicine* 317 (1987): 550–56.

5 S. B. Soumerai et al., "Effect of Medicaid Drug-Payment Limits on Admission to Hospitals and Nursing Homes," *New England Journal of Medicine* 325 (1991): 1072-77.

6 Evans, *Strained Mercy*, ch. 2.

7 C. D. Naylor, C. M. Levington, and S. Wheeler, "Queuing for Coronary Surgery During Severe Supply-Demand Mismatch in a Canadian Referral Centre: A Case Study of Implicit Rationing," *Social Science and Medicine* 37 (1993): 61-67.

8 C. D. Naylor, "Grey Zones of Clinical Practice: Some Limits to Evidence-Based Medicine," *Lancet* 345 (1995): 840-42.

9 J. E. Hux et al., "Are the Marginal Returns of Coronary Artery Surgery Smaller in High Rate Areas?" (submitted for publication, 1996).

10 C. D. Naylor, K. Sykora, and S. B. Jagkel, "Waiting for Coronary Artery Bypass Surgery: Population-Based Study of 8,517 Consecutive Patients in Ontario, Canada," *Lancet* 346 (1995): 1605-09.

11 C. M. Winslow et al., "The Appropriateness of Performing Coronary Artery Bypass Surgery," *Journal of the American Medical Association* 260 (1988): 505-9.

12 J. I. Williams et al., "The Burden of Waiting for Hip and Knee Replacements in Ontario," Working Paper no. 34, Institute for Clinical Evaluative Sciences, Toronto, 1995.

13 Evans, *Strained Mercy*, ch. 2.

14 V. Palda, personal communication.

15 E. Vayda, "Physicians in Health Care Management, Part 5: Payment of Physicians and Organization of Medical Services," *Canadian Medical Association Journal* 150 (1994): 1583-88; T. Bodenheimer and K. Grumbach, "Reimbursing

Physicians and Hospitals," *Journal of the American Medical Association* 272 (1994): 971–77.

16 J. Hurley and R. Card, "Global Physician Budgets as Common-Property Resources: Some Implications for Physicians and Medical Associations," *Canadian Medical Association Journal* 154 (1996): 1161–68.

Arthur Froese

The Power of the Physician: A Christian Perspective

Clothe yourselves with compassion, kindness, humility, gentleness and patience . . . whatever you do, whether in word or deed, do it all in the name of the Lord Jesus. — Colossians 3:12-17 (NIV)

A topic as broad as "The Power of the Physician" is an onerous one to condense. One approach would be to focus exclusively on power issues in the physician-patient relationship. However, we also wanted to discuss power as it pertains to other relationships in which the physician is involved, because this has been a much-neglected topic in the medical literature. Traditionally, physicians as a professional group have not recognized the power they have had over others, including nurses, office staff, and other paramedical professionals or students.

After some introductory remarks about the power of the physician, we will address power issues in the relationships between physicians and other professionals, including their staff and students. We will then deal with power in the physician-patient relationship. We also anticipated that the audience would include counsellors from a number of disciplines and will therefore say something about abuses of power in the counselling relationship. The concluding section will offer some general guidelines for avoiding misuse of power. Although we will frequently focus on sexual abuse, we do not want our audience to get the impression that that is all there is. Abuse of power can masquerade in many forms.

Physician Power
It is generally assumed that the relationship between physician and

patient will be one of benign caring, devoid of exploitation and abuse. Yet, the recognition that the physician-patient relationship has the potential for abuse and exploitation dates back many centuries—to a time before the Oath of Hippocrates. Richard Kluft has said that the oath "emphatically commands the physician to respect and protect the vulnerabilities of those to whom he or she attends. It demonstrates a recognition, across time and culture, of the tremendous power accorded to the physician by our society, and the potential for that power to be misused."[1] Indeed, within the oath, the power was considered to be so great that the sanction of God was invoked as part of the physician's covenant with the patient.

Despite its potential for misuse, the topic of power is one which is rarely considered by physicians themselves. For example, when we conducted a literature search on the topic of power, we encountered more than six hundred articles published in the past five years. However, the majority of these were written by nurses about their relative lack of power and ways in which this might be ameliorated. This was similar to Kluft's own computer search which "revealed a mere handful of references, mostly related to nursing journals' discussions of physicians abusing their power with nurses."[2]

What are the unique sources of power in the physician-patient relationship? The *first* of these comes to the physician through the *illness of the patient*. When we are ill, it is natural for us to become somewhat disconnected from the real world. However slightly ill we may be, we lose some of our sense of control through this loss of, or dispersion of, our connectedness with reality. A *second* source of power comes from the *specialized fund of knowledge* that the physician possesses. Such knowledge may be inaccessible or incomprehensible or both to the patient and thus tilts the power differential in favour of the physician. A *third* source of power comes to the physician through *social ascription* as in social or legal sanctions which allow the physician to prescribe drugs, determine one's competence, or even certify one, thus enforcing hospitalization against one's will. A *fourth* source of physician power comes from *dependency of the sick on the physician*. Patients expect the physician to respond to their needs. The greater the patient's neediness and the greater her degree of suffering, the greater will be her dependence on her physician. A *fifth* source of physician power comes from the *physician's sense of personal*

power and his/her status as a physician. A *sixth* source of physician
power comes from the *privilege accorded to the doctor to know* (see and
hear) what would normally be cloaked in privacy. These private
transactions between the physician and patient are predicated on
there being a significant level of trust in the relationship, specifically
trust by the patient of the physician.

How much abuse of physician power there may be will vary to
some extent with the nature of the physician-patient relationship.
Robert Veatch, in a 1972 *Hastings Center Report*, distinguished four
physician-patient relationship models.[3] In the *Engineering Model*, the
physician frequently behaves like an applied scientist. The physician
must be factual, divorced from all considerations of value, and simply present the patient with diagnosis, prognosis, and treatment options. The final decision-making is left completely up to the patient.
In this model questions of ethics and values are not entertained by
the physician. In Veatch's *Priestly Model* we encounter what is also
often called the paternalistic model. It reverses the Engineering
Model, so that in the Priestly Model it is the physician who decides
what constitutes benefit and harm. This model is exemplified by the
oft-used phrase, "Now, 'speaking-as-a-physician,' that is a risk I would
advise you not take." The locus of decision-making is taken from the
patient and placed in the physician's hands. In the *Collegial Model*,
the physician and patient are connected through common bonds,
seeing themselves as colleagues pursuing the common goal of eliminating the illness. Themes of trust and confidence play a most crucial role. There is an equality of dignity, respect, and value, but the
author himself asks whether there is, in fact, any real basis for the
assumption that the Collegial Model could apply to the physician-
patient relationship. In his final model, the *Contractual Model* the
differences in knowledge and power between the physician and patient are recognized. Veatch's Contractual Model attempts to com-
pensate for this power differential in terms of an assumed and sometimes explicit contractual perspective which enables both parties to
retain their dignity and moral authority. In this model if trust and
confidence are broken, then the contract is broken.

Trust in the Physician-Patient Relationship
Let us now take a closer look at trust and its role in the physician-

patient relationship. In his 1995 book, *The Illusion of Trust: Toward a Medical Theological Ethics in the Postmodern Age*, Edwin R. DuBose of Chicago says that it is clear that trust is indispensable when describing the patient-physician relationship and that there is little doubt that people generally trust physicians.[4] Traditionally the physician is the patient's fiduciary agent, whose sole obligation is to act in the patient's best interest. DuBose states further that, in recent times, there is a perception that physicians have other obligations that compete with their obligation to their patient. He feels that one price for the successes of technological biomedicine is the escalating financial costs of health care. Another price of this success is the erosion of trust in the physician-patient relationship. Trust is a basic ingredient in the clinical physician-patient encounter. This trust is most vulnerable when patients are ill.

Physicians' power, authority, and prestige reside in the image cultivated by them, that is, that physicians know as much as can be known about what they are doing and that they also are best informed about what is best for their patient. With the enormous advances in this technological age it is clear that even when doing their best, physicians often don't know what they are doing nor do they always know what is best for their patient. Consequently, many people are growing distrustful of physicians. The public attitude towards physicians has become one of distrust, cynicism, and suspicion.

The natural response to the absence of trust in relationships is for people to seek more direct control over these relationships. When this balance of power within relationships is upset, it is natural for the involved parties to seek to restore a more acceptable balance of power. Therefore, both parties tend to begin with efforts to preserve their individual power and autonomy in what has now become an adversarial relationship. In the physician-patient relationship, the patient may come to fear abuse and deception by the physician thus removing the unconditional trust that might once have been there. In response to this loss of trust, the physician may retreat to a defensive position pursuing self-interest. In the name of acting in the patient's best interest, a physician may act instead to preserve the profession's authority. In today's climate the danger lies in professionals retrenching and reverting back to previous structures of power and thus naturally sliding into adversarial relationships.

With the loss of trust in this postmodern age, concepts such as God, science, medicine, and principles of autonomy or justice may also be lost. DuBose says, "If there are no foundational truths to serve as the basis of our relations with one another, where once one could assume that the image of the physician represented trust, predictability, and accountability, we would seem to be left merely with relationships of mutual self-defense and self-interest."[5]

In an attempt to reassert its control over physicians, society has resorted to distrusting its physicians. David Mechanic suggests that this erosion of public trust is at least in part due to the profession's drift from its commitment to trustworthy behaviour and beneficence to a concentration on profit and prestige.[6] Leon Eisenberg has claimed that this present day disenchantment with physicians, "at a time when they can do more than ever in history to halt and repair the ravages of serious illness, probably reflects the perception by people that they are not being cared for."[7] The attempt to use distrust to balance the power between the public and the medical profession is reacted to by physicians with equal suspicion and distrust of the public. According to DuBose, in an attempt to "gain power and control of its art, the medical profession developed an organized structure, developed an institutional ideology, limited access to its ranks, and claimed 'status' as a profession acting in the best interest of its clients."[8]

DuBose goes on to suggest that there is a Christian solution to the public's loss of trust in its physicians. He suggests that it was originally a drift from Christian values and tradition that caused the loss of trust. In his opinion,

> in the broad, popular Christian tradition, the image of the transcendent creator God provides a central focus for a sense of meaning and reality. It is assumed that God exists or has reality distinct from and independent of human nature and our way of thinking about God. In the postmodern age, however, the relevancy of God to human life is an open question for many people. Once the notion of God-as-center is bracketed, the human community is thrown upon its own resources for identity and coherence.[9]

With the loss of trust and the loss of God as central in all relationships, there is now no foundational truth to serve as the basis upon which relationships hinge. According to DuBose, "we would seem to be left merely with relationships of mutual self-defense and self-interest . . . denial of God as central to human life and the elevation of humankind to centrality throws individuals into confrontation with other selves, and finally with the otherness within themselves."[10]

With recent progress in biomedical knowledge and technology, the already major physician-patient power differential has increased to the point of threatening the public. The public has reacted by asserting greater control over physicians through distrust, legislative constraints, and even litigation if necessary.

Physicians must therefore come to terms with the significant power differential that exists between them and their patients, other professionals, those who work for them, and students entrusted to them. The relationship that has evolved between the public and the medical profession is no longer one of unilateral dependence of the patient on the physician. As DuBose puts it so clearly, "The medical profession is in a mutually dependent relationship with the patient and also with the public that 'permits' or 'licenses' his or her practice, and gives to him the trust that is fundamental to his work (literally, the trust that allows the doctor 'to cut someone')."[11] DuBose goes on to state that

> if mutual trust is to exist in social relations, each person must be willing to surrender something of his or her self-control and accept the vulnerability that accompanies the dialectical structure of social existence. This surrender goes beyond contractual confidence, yet stops short of blind faith. It leads to the nature of trust and faith as *fides* and *fiducia* in a covenantal relationship.[12]

We physicians must come to recognize the interdependence that is necessary for an acceptable physician-patient relationship. DuBose puts it thus, "The person who acknowledges his or her dependency is better able to face the responsibility and obligations of the patient, who must relinquish some self-control to the doctor in trusting acceptance of the caring relationship. In the covenantal model, the doctor who gives care receives trust; the patient who gives trust receives care."[13]

In the Old Testament, the covenantal model is sometimes presented as a contract between people with God serving as a guarantor, for example, when Laban said to Jacob, "May the Lord keep watch between you and me when we are away from each other."[14] While such a covenantal approach is a good model for a Christian (or Jewish or Muslim) physician working with a patient of the same faith, it breaks down when the patient does not share the physician's values and beliefs. The development of strong collegial regulation of physicians represents a new covenant with a medical college serving as the guarantor. Such secular covenants depend on mutual faith in the College of Physicians and Surgeons to maintain a trustworthy relationship between physician and patient.

The Physician, Staff, Other Professionals, and Students

The training of physicians, beginning with their undergraduate work and continuing through medical school, internship, and residency, may contribute to the reaction many physicians have to their power status. In a brief paper published just over a year ago, "Some Musings on the Physician-God Syndrome,"[15] Arthur Schiff of Miami relates some interesting concepts. He tells an tired, old joke about the physician who dies and goes to heaven. Seeing a long line standing before St. Peter's desk, located just outside the pearly gates, he reasons that as a scientist and a physician, he should not have to wait in line. He hurries quickly to the head of the line and is informed by St. Peter that no special privileges are granted physicians or even Supreme Court Justices. Disgruntled, he stomps to the end of the line and prepares for a long wait. Just then, he sees a distinguished-looking man carrying a physician's bag hurry up to the pearly gates. This man is immediately buzzed into heaven by St. Peter. Once more the physician strides up to St. Peter and once more is told to return to the back of the line. St. Peter explains that it was God who hurried into Heaven and that God enjoys playing doctor every now and then.

Throughout our medical training the hierarchies are clear and we are repeatedly sent back to the end of the line after having climbed to the top—first as we climb to the top in our undergraduate years, and then as we enter medical school where we begin at the bottom again. An internship/residency program follows and we eventually become chief resident, but again we slip to the bottom of the line as we take up a junior staff position. Through the difficult climb to the top, according to Schiff, all the accoutrements the physician has garnered in this rocky and difficult climb take on an addictive quality. The system rewards us for being "better than" colleagues. There seems to be a tension between competence and superiority. This can lead to emotional patterns whereby we feel comfortable and secure when we are clearly superior to others in information, techniques, power, position, etc. As Schiff puts it, "the power of godhood can be as addictive as the power of drugs."[16] This power, once attained can lead to abuse and harassment of those less powerful. Therefore, many physicians, by the time they reach a staff position, will have experienced abuse and/or harassment from those above them on their way up the ladder. Despite Schiff's arguments, many other professionals go through a similar process, so this pattern is probably inadequate, in and of itself, to explain views on power.

In two studies of harassment and abuse reported by medical students in Canada and the United States, about half of medical students interviewed experienced some form of sexual harassment during their training. The experience in the Canadian study was somewhat lower than in the American study with 46% of women and 19% of men reporting sexual harassment during medical school. This is particularly unfortunate in the case of men where the abuse is likely to be perpetuated.[17]

Why is this? Why do physicians perpetuate such abuse? Karen Guise, in her Presidential address at the annual meeting of the Association for Academic Surgery in 1993, suggests that part of the problem is that there is an arrogance of power.[18] She goes on to state that this is often attributed to surgeons whose attitude is consistent with that of Donald Regan, former White House chief of Staff, when he stated, "I'm not arrogant. I just believe there's no human problem that couldn't be solved—if people would simply do as I tell 'em."[19] Speaking of surgeons, Guise continues, "We are guilty of denying our own failings. We become parochial and limited in our approach. We yell, scream, throw instruments, and act like children if we don't get our way or if a schedule cannot be changed to accommodate our needs."[20] She suggests that the distinction between self-confidence and arrogance can be subtle. As we shall elaborate later, we feel that pride is a significant trait that perpetuates abuse.

Several examples of abuse and harassment come to mind.

Case Study #1
A secretarial candidate interviewed for a job within a hospital. She was offered the job, but a few days later the Human Resources department indicated that she would not be taking the job. As it turned out, the secretary was so terrified of the anticipated reaction of her current physician boss that she would not discuss the possible transfer, even if accompanied by Human Resources staff. The fear was grounded in past experiences with this particular physician, which involved verbally and physically abusive behaviour.

The secretary continues to work in this unhappy situation, still unable to leave. Worse, the institutional regulations were such that no one felt they had the right to interfere, unless the victim initiated a complaint. Why is this? We know that such victims of harassment and abuse are often unable on their own of taking the necessary steps to get themselves out of such an abusive situation. We fail to recognize the parent-child nature of such relationships, and fail to recognize that it is *our*—everyone's—responsibility to lend our own power to victims of abuse.

Case Study #2
A senior resident was assisting in a delicate neuro-surgical procedure, and in the tension of the moment dropped a bone flap, much to the dismay of the neurosurgeon. Instead of being compassionate and understanding of the resident's unfortunate accident, the attending surgeon yelled at the resident and ordered him to stand in the corner, facing it for the rest of the procedure. The neurosurgeon in this case had a reputation of being bigoted, racist, and anti-Semitic. The resident feared that he would not get credit for years of Canadian training if he did not obey, and stood obediently in the corner for the three hours.

These may be extreme cases, but they are nonetheless true scenarios disguised somewhat to protect the innocent. Both of the examples described fall under what is called workplace harassment.

Such harassment or abuse is often related to gender or race. However, it may be part of a general pattern of bullying and badgering as well. What is meant by workplace harassment? Are such incidents not merely examples of personality clashes or polarization of viewpoints? Perhaps that is so in some cases where there is not a significant power differential between the involved individuals. However, if there is a significant power differential between them, the situation can easily evolve into harassment or abuse.

In their paper on workplace harassment, Simola and Parker point out that the Equal Employment Opportunity Commission in the United States and the Canadian Human Rights Act prohibit discrimination on specific grounds.[21] The Canadian Rights Act list of prohibitions includes race, national or ethnic origin, colour, religion, age, sex, marital status, family status, mental or physical disability, and pardoned conviction.[22] According to the 1993 Canadian Human Rights Commission guidelines, harassment will be deemed to have occurred if, "a reasonable person ought to have known that the behaviour was unwelcome."[23] The grounds for harassment in the guidelines of both the American and Canadian legislation deal with characteristics of the victim over which the victim has no control—such as race, colour, sex, age, etc.—which are referred to as "ascribed" characteristics. Everyone, be they a perpetrator or a victim, also possesses non-ascribed or "achieved" characteristics such as attained level of education, professional title, or level of income.[24] In workplace settings, "achieved" characteristics often contribute to the power differential between perpetrator and victim. As mentioned these can include educational level attained, professional title, or income level. Traditionally, physicians by virtue of their increased status have greater power than do nurses, technicians, psychologists, social workers, occupational, and physiotherapists, to mention a few.

The Canadian Human Rights Commission gives guidelines to provide protection and recourse to those suffering from racial or sexual harassment and the like. It does not protect or offer recourse to individuals who are bullied or abused by those with more powerful "achieved" characteristics. Moreover, Employment Standards Acts do not, at present, protect employees from abuse due to power differentials based on "achieved" characteristics.

A model of workplace harassment requiring five necessary conditions for harassment to occur is offered by Simola and Parker.[25] These five necessary conditions are:

1. A dyad of people in interaction
2. A power differential between them
3. An abuse of power by the perpetrator
4. Direct hurt to the victim
5. Unresponsiveness of the perpetrator to adequate feedback

From a Christian perspective, the teachings of Matthew 18:15-18 are appropriate here. We shall refer to this more specifically later.

Hurt for the victim

> can result from a number of experiences which are disrespectful, demeaning, or offensive. This behavior threatens the physical, emotional, spiritual, or cognitive well-being of the victim. It may also jeopardize the victim's professional credibility. Hurt is subjectively defined, and could involve a broad spectrum of experiences, ranging from anger or frustration right through to signs and symptoms of depression, anxiety, or post-traumatic stress.[26]

Based on previous research by others, Simola and Parker list four categories of workplace harassment.[27] The categories are not mutually exclusive, thus victims may experience one or more at the hands of the same perpetrator. *First*, they mention intimidation or threats, which involve the use of implied or overt verbal threats such as a loud voice, specific looks, physical gestures, or actions which instil fear or uncertainty in another. A *second* technique is that of professional isolation. The perpetrator, through the use of prohibitions or censuring, attempts to maintain control over the victims by keeping them separate from their colleagues or other sources of support. A *third* technique of perpetrators is to make unreasonable or unethical demands of their victims. These may include attempts to coerce victims into completing tasks which are not part of their job description or which ought not reasonably be required of them. The *fourth* technique is what Simola and Parker describe as a flagrant disrespect for and undermining of the victim's professional credibility. This may involve public ridicule of the victim's professional skills through unfounded criticism and untrue assertions which have no basis in scholarly theory or research, but which are used merely to silence or demean the victim. It may also involve the perpetrator blaming the victim for the perpetrator's own errors.

We do not want to imply that those who are guilty of these forms of harassment are the same individuals who would approach their patients sexually. We are not aware of studies examining the profiles of those who are guilty of harassment. However, from our personal experience in observing those who do harass, and hearing of them, we would suggest that many harassers are intensely insecure and immature individuals who suffer from feelings of inadequacy and who have a major pride problem. According to Leanne Payne in *Restoring the Christian Soul,* "Feelings of inadequacy and inferiority (like those of presumption and superiority), no matter from what psychological injury they stem, are ultimately rooted in pride."[28] Emotionally they are fearful little children who are intensely insecure and who feel incompetent to such a degree, that their pride will not allow them to admit these fears even to themselves. This is the pride component which plays an important role in the dynamics of those who harass others. C. S. Lewis, in *Mere Christianity,* calls pride *the great sin* and says of it:

> There is one vice of which no man in the world is free;
> which every one in the world loathes when he sees it in
> someone else; and of which hardly any people . . . ever
> imagine that they are guilty of themselves . . . the proud
> man, even when he has got more than he can possibly
> want, will try to get still more just to assert his power.[29]

If you cannot admit your inadequacies, you must account for your perceived failures somehow. Since you do not have the where-with-all to "elevate" yourself you deal with the situation by demeaning and "lowering" those about you. Lewis says, "A proud man is always looking down on things and people."[30]

These individuals are intensely threatened by competent people around them, particularly peers and colleagues. Therefore, they have a need to "perform" to an audience to reassure themselves of their own competence. Thus, they often harass their victim with others present, almost as a warning to the onlookers, that they dare not show their competence or they will be equally harassed or abused.

One way of disarming the harasser is to play to their pride, telling them how wonderful they are. However, this is a very temporary solution, and one that comes at great personal cost to the victim.

Long-term solutions for such perpetrators requires intense therapy to deal with the underlying fears, inadequacies, and immaturity. To deal with the pride requires a spiritual solution, and this is usually difficult if not impossible without a major spiritual awakening. In Leanne Payne's words: "I steadfastly and consistently denied throughout my life the little girl in me who would admit her fear of rejection and exposure, inadequacy and inferiority. . . . Therefore, I had to confess pride and receive forgiveness for it."[31]

Simola and Parker address a further issue that merits mention. This has to do with abuses of power that may occur as the institutional "administration" re-victimizes the one already abused:

> It is important to note that administrative responses to complaints of harassment might well follow and support the existing structures of power within the organization. Since the existing power relationships were necessary to enable the harassment, the support of these power structures could potentially re-victimize the complainant, or bolster the extant harassment.[32]

For example, complainants might experience isolation if given instructions not to involve their union or consult a lawyer. The victim is thus re-victimized by administration and may not act in his or her best interest out of fear of the consequences, and not contact their union or lawyer.

The Physician-Patient Relationship

Abuses of power by physicians is a topic that Richard Kluft has covered in fair detail.[33] He begins with a section entitled, "Physicians Acting as Agents of Social Control." In this section he points to five identifiable steps by which the Nazis carried out the principle of "life unworthy of life," including acts such as sterilization, killing of "impaired" children, killing of "impaired" adults (mostly patients in mental hospitals), impaired inmates of concentration and extermination camps and finally to mass killing, mostly of Jews. Some see liberal abortion laws and beginning trends towards euthanasia, and artificial methods of reproduction as part of this particular "slippery slope" toward abuse of power. Kluft then goes on to discuss "Physicians Subverting Medical Rights and Prerogatives for Illicit

Purposes," including the performance of unnecessary procedures and surgeries. In his next section, "Physicians Exploiting the Power of their Profession to Gratify Personal Needs Related to Their Neurotic or Character Difficulties" Kluft refers both to the narcissistic need for the physician to be totally in control and the need to be perceived as perfect. Under "Physicians Causing Patients to Receive Less Than Optimal Care" he refers to physician behaviours that seem to reflect what in psychotherapeutic terms would be called countertransference. In "Physicians Allowing the Subversion of Their Medical Judgment," he expresses concern about new concepts such as "managed care" and their possible effects on medical care. What is best for the patient and what is palatable to those who hold the purse-strings is an interface that is subject to much potential abuses. Two further areas of concern include, "Physicians Causing the Delivery of Less than Optimal Care" and "The Physician's Role in the Dehumanizing Medical Care." His final three sections deal with physicians as perpetrators of sexual misconduct, the consequences for patients of such abuse, and the treatment of patients who have been sexually abused by physicians.

The final report of the Ontario Task Force on sexual abuse of patients released November 25, 1991, considers sexual impropriety or sexual violation to include, but not be limited to, the following:

- Watching a patient dress or undress instead of providing privacy
- Deliberately making sexual comments about a patient's body or under clothing
- Making sexualized or sexually-demeaning comments to a patient
- Criticism of the patient's sexual orientation
- Making comments about potential sexual performance unless consultation was to discuss sexual issues
- Making a request to date
- Subjecting a patient to an examination in the presence of medical students or other parties without explicit consent
- Requesting details of sexual history or sexual likes/dislikes when not indicated relative to presenting problem
- Initiating conversation regarding the sexual problems, preferences, or fantasies of the physician

◆ All contact with genitals without use of gloves.[34]

One might rightly ask, how often do such abuses occur? We do not know because we do not even have quantitative Canadian studies identifying the incidence of sexual abuse by physicians, let alone other forms of abuse. American self-report surveys place the incidence of sexual or erotic contact (defined as behaviours primarily intended to arouse or satisfy sexual desire) or sexual intercourse with patients by physicians at 5 to 13% of physicians. Between 5 and 7.2% specifically acknowledge engaging in sexual intercourse with patients.[35] A relatively recent Canadian study found that 8% of Ontario women reported sexual harassment or abuse by doctors. On average, only 40% of those who acknowledged that they were sexually abused ever reported what happened to them.[36]

Who are the physicians who sexually abuse their patients? The *first group* of physicians at serious risk are those with *role identity problems.* Included are physicians who, for their own difficulties, find themselves in an emotionally depleted state, for example as might happen following disruption of a personal relationship or illness. Physicians in this state are at risk of allowing a role reversal to develop between them and their patient. The patient in such a relationship may be seduced into a role of rescuing the physician. Alternatively, the physician may represent intimacies as sex therapy. Another danger signal may be exemplified when positive transference is exploited and the physician takes expressions of positive feelings at face value and responds to them. Role identity problems can also come about when the physician first creates and then exploits his patient's exaggerated dependency. It is important to note that as Christian Physicians we are not immune from these temptations or stressors.[37] A *second group* of difficulties come about when the physician uses *physical or emotional force* in an abusive way. Forceful sexual or other advances and threats or intimidation to procure sexual satisfaction are examples. This may also include claims of true love for the patient on the part of the doctor, or claims that the situation "just got out of hand." Another scenario may come about when the physician is convinced that the situation between him and the patient is a special one. A *third group* of risk factors we have called *psychopathic scenarios* and include the physician who uses drugs in the service of seduction or blackmail in the form of threats of disclosing sensitive confidential information. This latter group are extremely narcissistic, self-centred individuals, lacking of conscience, and driven by their animalistic desires. They are what M. Scott Peck identifies as basically evil in his book entitled *People of the Lie*.[38]

Who are the victims? In many cases it is the average patient who becomes a victim of the power differential. However, victims of past abuse are more powerless and hence particularly vulnerable. Often these patients put a great deal into maintaining relationships at the expense of their own needs and interests. Some have learned, through early conditioning, that physical affection and physical touching are the only ways of relating, and may feel that this represents true love. Because they blame themselves for what is happening to them, they keep the information to themselves out of shame and therefore do not disclose the abuse. They may have problems assessing interpersonal relationships and have difficulty judging when they are being used or mistreated. They may even feel that they deserve what is happening to them. Their cognition may be impaired so that they are unable to assess an abusive situation and fail to see the abusive nature of it. Therefore they may fail to run from situations when others with better judgment would. These individuals easily become dependent in relationships and feel that they must maintain the relationship at all cost. Unfortunately, perpetrators have an uncanny ability to recognize these individuals.

In Richard Kluft's assessment they are easily re-victimized. One profile to which he refers is "the sitting duck syndrome."[39] This includes patients who, due to past abuse, are distrustful individuals who are generally fearful of medical encounters and find medical settings intimidating. They therefore frequently delay seeking help for any reason. When they do attend they tend to be uneasy and suspicious, often taking a defensive and angry stance when dealing with any authority figures, but especially physicians. They lack self-confidence and manifest low self-esteem. If sexual exploitation is part of their history, they show signs of Post Traumatic Stress Disorder complete with flashbacks, nightmares, intense fear, hypervigilance, exaggerated startle response, and self-mutilating behaviours.

Physician Power and Psychotherapy (Counselling)

Nowhere is the potential for the power differential greater than in the therapist-psychotherapy patient relationship. The *first* reason for this is transference, that is, those positive or negative feelings the patient experiences towards the therapist, which derive from significant emotional relationships from the past, that are now transferred to the therapist. These feelings and opinions patients have towards their physician may have relatively little to do with the here-and-now experience, but through transference the power of that physician may be amplified several times. Transference puts the therapist in a position of great power. When a patient's feelings take on a sexual nature, the opportunity for abuse is great unless treatment boundaries are set by the physician and adhered to. A *second* problem is that in the psychotherapy relationship, the therapist is often dealing with the most vulnerable patients. The patient may be a depressed individual whose cognition is slowed, whose judgment may be impaired, and whose feelings of hopelessness and helplessness prevent her from recognizing what may be in her best self interest. Such individuals invariably feel totally disempowered and are unable to defend against abusive treatment. In addition, many will feel much guilt and view themselves as deserving of punishment and abuse.

Alternatively, one may be dealing with an individual who is perplexed, whose thinking processes are disturbing to self and others, and who may be becoming increasingly suspicious and experiencing other symptoms of early schizophrenia. Voices may be heard that others seem not to hear. Comments made over the radio or television may be inferred to have special personal meaning. Such a patient in a counselling situation may over-interpret the therapist's comments, looks, or gestures and thus responds in a sexualized way in return. Such sexualized advances, when not understood in the context of transference, may overwhelm the inexperienced therapist who may fail to set and enforce appropriate treatment boundaries and then fall into allowing some sexual acting out on the part of the patient, or even on the part of the therapist.

Unfortunately the most vulnerable are the patients who have a history of abuse in their background, be it verbal, physical, or sexual abuse. Such individuals are even more vulnerable when they have also been victimized by professionals from whom they have sought help. Of those who are unfortunate enough to be incest survivors, 23% (almost one in four) who go for help end up being abused sexually by their "helpers."[40]

Again we see the parallel with the parent-child relationship. Richard Kluft has said, "To the extent that the patient is dependent on someone for his or her well-being who has superior knowledge and power and who is perceived as the embodiment of the parental omnipotence encountered and depended on by a young child, the doctor-patient relationship is a parent-child relationship in form and structure."[41]

Psychotherapy (counselling) is an activity that many underestimate. All too often, one encounters the phrase, "anyone can do it," in reference to therapy. Consequently, many who take on the task of therapist are ill trained and lacking in experience and thus fail to recognize important issues such as transference, counter-transference, resistance, etc. They therefore fail to set safeguards as appropriate and consistent therapeutic boundaries.

Case Study #3
This victim, a young woman in her mid twenties with an MA in psychology sought help for anxiety and depression. As a young child she was abused by a male baby sitter. During college she sought help from the University Health Services. Under the pretext of therapy, her therapist seduced her into a sexual relationship that lasted two years. A few years later, when she began her second course of therapy with her new therapist, that relationship also began to be sexualized when she verbally expressed a desire to hug her new therapist. Fortunately, the resident therapist (working under the guidance of an astute and experienced supervisor) was able to keep the boundaries of therapy clear. The desire to hug the therapist became the topic of much important material in subsequent sessions.

In most provinces, a great deal of psychotherapy, both brief and long term, is practised by non-psychiatrist physicians. Due to the high cost of private therapy by non-physician therapists, many patients deliberately seek out physician therapists who are covered by Medicare. While some physician-therapists seek training and supervision in psychotherapy, many do not. The level of training and skill therefore varies widely between physician-therapists as it does for non-physician therapists. According to the *Ontario Task Force* on sexual abuse, "many physicians believe that little or no special training is required to do psychotherapy."[42] Yet, it is well known that, "providing effective therapy requires a high level of skill and training just as other medical specialties, such as surgery or pediatrics, do."[43]

Unfortunately, most undergraduate medical training programs have failed to teach student physicians how to recognize symptoms of sexual abuse. Until recently, training in this area was totally inadequate in most psychiatric training programs. It would be difficult to imagine that medical, paediatric, or surgical programs did better. The task force found troubling attitudes throughout its process. Some of the troubling attitudes include the following:

- The tendency to blame victims for the abuse, rather than realizing that because the physician has more power in the relationship, it is always the physician's responsibility not to abuse, no matter what the circumstances.
- The tendency to believe that women and children lie about sexual abuse, instead of recognizing that most abuse is never reported, and that false reports, while not impossible, are rare.
- The belief that the patient is in a position to consent to the abuse, and that if she did so, sexual abuse had not taken place.
- The belief that sexual abuse is probably not that harmful, since physical force and violence may not have been present.
- The belief that reports of sexual abuse by patients must be due to misunderstanding by patients of procedures that are entirely appropriate.[44]

Sometimes therapy techniques and procedures are used by therapists Who do things to patients that are abusive, but are not recognized as such by the therapists. The same technique may have been appropriate for another patient, and not experienced as abusive.

Case Study #4

An eighteen-year-old, timid, insecure, and passive woman sought therapy from a holistic medical practitioner. She sought help for symptoms of depression, anxiety, and homicidal impulses towards parents that she could not understand. In the background was a history of parental neglect, but no known parental abuse. As a child, she was witness to sexual abuse of a friend by several adolescent boys and a teenager exposing himself to her on her way home from school. When she was a young teen, a young adult male was caught on a ladder looking into her second storey bedroom window. In therapy her physician therapist soon identified sexual anxieties. Once an intense dependency on him had developed, in his efforts to help her, he "forced" her to buy and discuss pornographic magazines as part of a deconditioning process. When she hesitated to follow through he threatened to stop therapy. By now she was far too dependent and could not refuse to comply. Further in therapy he would get her to lie on a mat on his office floor and as part of his 'touch therapy' would lie on top of her, presumably again to decondition her of her "fear of men." Such therapy for an abuse survivor can only be seen as re-victimization.

How to Prevent Harassment

Many physicians are aware of the power they possess as well as the potential that exists for misuse of that power, yet some do abuse it. It is clear that in the past physicians have not been adequately taught about harassment, abuse, power differentials, etc. Society is now better informed about these issues and it is the responsibility of every physician also to be fully informed. This is especially so with respect to sexual abuse. Physicians as a professional group must also become better informed about the hurt and damage harassment can cause. We must learn how we can avoid harassing others, and how best to protect patients from harassment by others. *Education is the key.*[45] However, we must also be receptive learners.

It is not within the scope of this paper to give a long list of specific guidelines, since the *Ontario Task Force* has done this. You can refer to its report for details. We will list only some of the highlights as follows:

1. Learn about power and its dynamics, especially as it relates to physicians and patients, but also as it relates to physicians and others.
2. Become informed on the issue; know what harassment and abuse are.
3. Become informed of the magnitude of the problem and its consequences to victims.
4. Learn strategies for recognizing, confronting, and treating

abuse by colleagues and how to report suspicion of abuse by colleagues.

5. Learn how to recognize and treat victims of past abuse sensitively.

6. Set and enforce appropriate treatment boundaries for yourself, your patients, your staff, your junior colleagues, your students, other non-medical professionals, etc.

7. If you are concerned that you might be at risk of harassing or abusing others, get help for yourself before it happens. Learn how to recognize the signs in your own behaviour.

8. Enlist your patients' help by making posters and brochures on the topic readily available to them in your office.

9. Through a compassionate and caring attitude inform your patients of their right to say "no"; their right to ask questions; their right to understand as they are able what is happening to them and their body at every stage of treatment; their right to report harassment and abuse and how to do it.

10. If you have reason to believe that you may have harassed or abused someone you do not know as a fellow Christian, you should seek the advice of the CMPA. Trying to resolve the issue according to principles set out in Matthew 18 may not be a valid first step, but will depend on the individual situation.

11. If you have reason to believe you may have harassed or abused a fellow Christian, then Matthew 18 definitely applies. That is, "If your brother sins against you, go and show him his fault, just between the two of you. If he listens to you, you have won your brother over. But if he will not listen, take one or two others along, so that 'every matter may be established by the testimony of the two or three witnesses.' If he refuses to listen to them, tell it to the church; and if he refuses to listen even to the church, treat him as you would a pagan or a tax collector" (NIV).

If you should find yourself, a colleague, or a patient a victim of harassment or abuse, the guidelines spelled out by Simola and Parker are valuable.[46] Their definition of harassment and their recommendations are consistent with a Matthew 18 procedure.

There was a time when the physician could pursue medicine in the context of a covenant involving the patient, the physician, and

God. This time may be gone for ever, but is certainly not present now. The new covenant in its place typically involves a rather powerful college. Besides avoiding being an abuser, there are at least two things that the Christian physician can do out of faith on behalf of the patient. One is to struggle to sustain the relevant college as a true covenanting body that sustains and sanctions the caring relationship between physician and patient. This is a task of continuing maintenance, not an effort that can be done and be complete. The second is to borrow an understanding from the Shaker faith. For the Shaker, his or her work was an act of worship, whatever the task.[47] The classic Shaker chair is a thing of beauty, function, and sacrifice because the maker was worshipping God in the making of the chair. As a caregiver, you can worship God in your acts of caring. The patient may be of any faith or no faith at all. The act of worship is between you and God, and in that act of worship you provide, as an act of sacrifice, your very best care. If you do that with honesty, intelligence, and love, you can't go too far wrong.

Summary

It is generally assumed that the relationship between the physician and the patient will be one of benign caring. We have pointed out the imbalance of power that exists in the relationship. Power is accorded the physician through:

1. The patient's loss of connectedness with reality when ill
2. The physician's specialized knowledge
3. Specific social and legal sanctions
4. Dependent needs of the ill
5. The physician's status
6. Access to privileged information

We have identified the important role trust plays in the physician-patient relationship. We have said that the erosion of trust in the relationship has moved the relationship into the adversarial arena, and that this shift has transferred further power to the physician. We have also emphasized the need for physicians to come to terms with the power differential and have identified possible physician-patient models that could enable both the physician and the patient to retain their own dignity and moral authority.

In the section on relationships with other professionals, staff, and students, we focused on harassment. This can be subtle and on the surface could be construed as a mere personality clash, were it not for the significant power differential. We have said that there are five necessary conditions for workplace harassment to take place:

1. A dyad
2. A power differential
3. Illegitimate use of that power
4. Hurt experience by the victim
5. An unresponsive perpetrator

We have said the techniques employed by the perpetrator include:

1. Intimidation or threats
2. Professional isolation
3. Unreasonable or unethical demands
4. Disrespect for and undermining of victim's professional credibility

With reference to physician-patient relationships, the focus was on sexual abuse issues, but the power the physician possesses puts the physician at significant risk to abuse in non-sexual ways as well. After several examples we reviewed the profile of the physician who sexually abuses patients and what are the danger signs. We also reviewed typical profiles for the victims of sexual abuse.

In the last section, we have said that the therapist-patient relationship is unique in that the power differential is compounded by a further weakened patient. We have pointed out that transference is a special power enhancing process and cautioned against thinking that anyone can do therapy. We have also outlined some points that can serve as guidelines for preventing misuse of power.

Notes

[1] R. P. Kluft, "The Physician as Perpetrator of Abuse," *Primary Care* 20 (1993): 459–80.

[2] Ibid., 462.

[3] R. M. Veatch, "Models for Ethical Medicine in a Revolutionary Age," *The Hastings Center Report* 2, no. 3 (1972): 5–7

[4] E. R. DuBose, *The Illusion of Trust: Toward A Medical Theological Ethics in the Postmodern Age* (Boston: Kluwer Academic Publishers, 1995), 34–37.

[5] Ibid., 10.

[6] D. Mechanic, "Public Perceptions of Medicine," *New England Journal of Medicine*

312 (1985): 181–83.

7   L. Eisenberg, "The Search for Care," *Daedalus* 106 (1977): 238.

8   DuBose, 40.

9   Ibid., 82.

10 Ibid., 85–87.

11 Ibid., 119.

12 Ibid.

13 Ibid., 122.

14 Genesis 31:49 (NIV).

15 A. F. Schiff, "Some Musings on the Physician-God Syndrome," *Archives of Family Medicine* 4 (1995): 193–94.

16 Ibid., 194.

17 T. M. Wolf et al., "Perceived Mistreatment and Attitude Change by Graduating Medical Students: A Retrospective Study," *Medical Education* 25 (1991): 182–90; R. Moscarello, K. J. Margittai, and M. Rossi, "Differences in Abuse Reported by Female and Male Canadian Medical Students," *Canadian Medical Association Journal* 150 (1994): 357–63.

18 K. S. Guice, "Power," presidential address, *Journal of Surgical Research* 56 (1994): 479–83.

19 Ibid., 481.

20 Ibid.

21 S. K. Simola and K. C. H. Parker, "Non-ascriptive Workplace Harassment: A Psychologists' Guide for Ethical and Effective Resolution" (unpublished paper, 1996).

22 Canadian Human Rights, c.H-6 R.S.C. (1985).

23 Canadian Human Rights Commission, *Harassment: What It Is and What to Do About It* (Ottawa: Minister of Supply and Services, 1993, brochure).

24 M. Spencer, *Foundations of Modern Sociology* (Scarborough, Ont.: Prentice Hall, 1981), 248–49.

25 Simola and Parker, 14.

26 Ibid., 17–18.

27 Ibid., 21–26.

28 L. Payne, *Restoring the Christian Soul Through Healing Prayer: Overcoming the Three Great Barriers to Personal and Spiritual Completion in Christ* (Wheaton, Ill.: Crossway Books, 1991), 96.

29 C. S. Lewis, *Mere Christianity*, (London: Fontana Books, 1952), 106.

30 Ibid., 108.

31 Payne, 96.

32 Simola and Parker, 34.

33 Kluft, 462–75.

[34] The College of Physicians and Surgeons of Ontario, An Independent Task Force Commissioned by the College of Physicians and Surgeons of Ontario [or CPSO], *The Final Report of the Task Force on Sexual Abuse of Patients* (Toronto, 1991), 46–47.

[35] Ibid., 13.

[36] Ibid., 82.

[37] G. Del Begio, "Doctor-Patient Sexual Abuse," *Focus* (March 1994): 15–19.

[38] M. S. Peck, *People of the Lie: The Hope for Healing Human Evil* (New York: Simon and Schuster, 1983), 69–77.

[39] Kluft, 474.

[40] J. Frenken and B. Von Stolk, "Incest Victims: Inadequate Help by Professions," *International Journal of Child Abuse and Neglect* (1990): 253–63.

[41] Kluft, 461.

[42] CPSO, 116.

[43] Ibid.

[44] Ibid., 120–21.

[45] The University of Toronto has instituted an educational program at both the undergraduate and postgraduate levels. Gail Erlick Robinson and Donna E. Stewart report on this program in a two part series published by the *Canadian Medical Association Journal*. Cf. G. E. Robinson and D. E. Stewart, "A Curriculum on Physician-Patient Sexual Misconduct and Teacher-Learner Mistreatment, Part 1: Content," *Canadian Medical Association Journal* 154 (March 1996): 643–649; Robinson and Stewart, "A Curriculum on Physician-Patient Sexual Misconduct and Teacher-Learner Mistreatment, Part 2: Teaching Method," *Canadian Medical Association Journal* 154 (April 1996): 1021–25.

[46] Simola and Parker, 30–36.

[47] K. Newman and S. Abell, "The Shakers' Brief Eternity," *National Geographic* 176, no. 3 (1989): 302–25.

Joseph L. Soria

Chastity in the Practice of Medicine

"Walk by the Spirit, and do not gratify the desires of the flesh. . . . Now the works of the flesh are plain: fornication, impurity, licentiousness . . . envy drunkenness, carousing, and the like. I warn you, as I warned you before, that those who do such things shall not inherit the kingdom of God."[1] We open our talk on "Chastity in the Practice of Medicine" with these words of Paul to the Galatians. The reason for doing so is important: we are going to deal with a subject very relevant not only at a human and professional level, but also necessary if one wishes to follow Our Lord Jesus Christ and so enter into the Eternal Kingdom.

One question which needs to be stated clearly from the outset is that there is no such a thing as an autonomous professional medical ethic, neither in sexual matters nor in any other field. The doctor is not exempted from the general moral law, but is subject to it, like everyone else. Not even the real or alleged needs of medical practice can legitimize immoral behaviour: "Why not do evil that good may come of it?" some people may argue. If we doctors are supposed to help people to recover their health, why not use all the means available, forgetting about prohibitions or limits of a religious nature? The answer was provided by St. Paul two thousand years ago in the letter to the Romans:[2] because those who advocate this are wrongly subordinating inferior goods to superior ones and—the Apostle says—"their condemnation is just." It is untenable for a physician to retort that what is motivated by medical needs cannot be judged by the ordinary standards of human behaviour, maintaining that things which are evil in social life can be justified in the medical field. It is, of course, true that surgical incisions, the unconsciousness following general anaesthesia, the use of drugs, etc., are a justifiable component of medical techniques and approach, while these same things must be rejected as immoral in ordinary human behaviour and relationships. But deeds which are evil in themselves never can be rendered good for any human reason. It will never be morally permissible to kill a person for the purpose of obtaining organs or tissues for transplantation into another person. It can never be right to recommend a lecherous type of living, with the intention of healing a patient from his depression.

In fact the particular needs or circumstances of medical practice do not find their origin in an autonomous set of moral standards, but in the application of general moral principles to specific tasks and circumstances.

One of the challenges that medical practice faces today is related to the misinterpretation of the nature of sex in our society. We are living and working in a hedonistic culture which seeks to separate sexuality from all objective moral norms. Often sex is seen as a mere diversion and a consumer good, to the point of justifying a kind of idolatry of the sexual instinct, with the powerful complicity of the means of social communication. Even the word *chastity* is either ignored or ridiculed as an oddity belonging to a supposed dark age. The real as well as the etymological kinship between chastity and chastisement is obvious, and therefore chastity is looked upon as something stern and austere; but this facade must not hide the beauties and riches of the loveable and royal building behind. That is why, before going further into our subject, we should devote some attention to the concept of chastity itself.

What Is Chastity?

The *Oxford American Dictionary* defines chastity as the condition of being chaste, i.e., not having sexual intercourse except with the person to whom one is married. I think that we are faced here with a very narrow understanding of chastity, and, needless to say, this is not going to be the way of dealing with our subject today. Just to mention one example, we clearly could not designate as chaste a physician who, though not engaging in sexual intercourse, indulges in all sorts of sexual activity with a patient.

In the larger *Oxford International Dictionary* the word *chastity* is also defined in connection with the word *chaste*. But *chaste* is now presented as having five different meanings, namely:

1. Pure from unlawful sexual intercourse, or continent, or virtuous
2. Celibate, single
3. Morally pure or innocent
4. Decent, free from indecency or offensiveness
5. Chastened, restrained from all excess

In this paper, we will consider all these meanings together, except meaning two (*celibate, single*), for obvious reasons.

In a broad manner, chastity may therefore be defined as the virtue which regulates human behaviour in connection with the sexual drive. It is a form of temperance, and consequently linked to self-control and sobriety. Sin caused division and disharmony in our nature, and, as St. Augustine put it sixteen centuries ago, "It is through chastity that we are gathered together and led back to the unity from which we were fragmented into multiplicity."[3] Chastity is often confused with modesty, though the latter is properly a circumstance or a complement of chastity. Modesty protects the inner sanctuary of a person.[4] It is born with the awakening consciousness of being a subject. It inspires one's choice of clothing. It keeps silence or reserve where there is evident risk of unhealthy curiosity. It is discreet. It protests against the voyeuristic explorations of the human body.

When the reasons for chastity are merely human, chastity remains at a natural level. When the motives of chastity are discovered in the light of faith in Jesus and incorporated into one's life, we can talk about Christian chastity, which is precisely the approach I am going to follow in this paper.

Allow me to repeat again that chastity is related to all sexual acts and behaviour which have a sexual implication, and not only to intercourse. In fact, when we are referring to a sexual act in the context of morality, we imply "any act whatsoever—whether thought, word, or deed—in which someone intends, either as an end in itself or as a means to some other end, to bring about or maintain sexual arousal and/or to cause incomplete or complete sexual satisfaction, whether in himself or herself, in another, or both."[5] Notice that, as happens in most precise definitions, poetry is absent when reason and logic are present. But notice also that in this comprehensive and articulate definition there is much food for thought. It somehow provides us with a standard for an honest and deep examination of conscience, because it confronts us with very private aspects of our life. I am referring to intimate thoughts or desires, secret motivations, selfish attitudes perhaps covered with glossy pseudo-scientific jargon, alleged principles which are not principles but the consequence of greed or peer pressure, etc. All these things, precisely because they do not reach the level of exterior or public deeds, cannot be scrutinized by anybody but ourselves—and God. And these are the main things which need to be analyzed in our inner self today. In a certain manner it is very easy to be considered a decent and chaste person by others; but this alone would be a rather silly goal: "there is nothing hid, except to be made manifest; nor is anything secret, except to come to light."[6] The important target is to be chaste in the eyes of the Lord, even if, in most cases, the fruit of chastity is not the purity of innocence but the purification of repentance: "your Father who sees in secret will reward you."[7]

But, we may ask ourselves, why is our sexuality (and therefore chastity) important to God? Is God equally concerned with our digestion, our kidney function, or any other bodily operation? I will return later to the specific anthropological dimensions of human sexuality and therefore of chastity. For the time being let us fix our attention on a more generic answer: chastity is important because unchastity—or lust—first and foremost violates God's will: "You shall not commit adultery."[8] It could be added that if any sin, being idolatrous self-love, is contrary to God's love, lust is specifically auto-idolatrous. "God is love,"[9] St. John teaches, and unchaste behaviour subordinates authentic love to sexual drive and pleasure, even if very often today love is trivialized and presented as the excuse for any sexual misconduct. A thorough discussion about the different kinds and levels of love would be very interesting, but would take us away from our subject.

From time to time you may read some superficial and ignorant criticisms of Christian chastity, wrongly identifying it with prudery, aversion to pleasure, horror of the flesh, and the like. Some people even try to justify their opposition by hastily assembling some quotes from the Bible, especially those from St. Paul, rejecting the "works of the flesh."[10] They seem to imply that Saint Paul is preaching a sort of

Manichean anthropological dualism, whereas, on the contrary, Pauline dualism is ascetical. In fact the "flesh," as Saint Paul used the term most of the time, refers, ironically, not to our bodies but to fallen nature. "Carnal" is not "bodily," or "material," because there are "carnal spirits." The "carnal" spirit is intemperate, the one that devours things for itself and refuses to make them an oblation to God. "The carnal spirit is cruel, egocentric, avaricious, gluttonous, and lecherous, and as such is fevered, restless, and divided. The spiritual man, on the other hand, is the man who both knows what flesh is for and can enter into its amplitude. The lecher, for example, supposes that he knows more about love than the virgin or the continent man. He knows nothing. Only the virgin and the faithful spouse know what love is about."[11]

I was saying that we are presently immersed in a culture in which sex has become a commodity. We are bombarded with numerous by-products of this frivolous approach, and now, as in previous times, chastity is not easy. However, we must add right away that it is not impossible, because divine grace empowers every Christian to pursue chastity and attain it. Of itself, the sexual drive does not express love; it is no more communicative than any other biological drive, like hunger or thirst. That is why, even within marriage, sexual activity must convey genuine love, in such a way that, unless freely chosen for the sake of the common benefit, marital intercourse cannot express and nurture unselfish love. Notice that chastity doesn't condemn human sexuality or sexual pleasure in themselves. It could not be otherwise, since both are the result of the divine will: "God created man in his own image . . . male and female he created them. And God blessed them, and God said to them, 'Be fruitful and multiply.'"[12] What chastity aims at is the successful integration of sexuality within the person, and thus the inner unity of man in his bodily and spiritual being. As history teaches, "insofar as Christian piety strives to detach itself from physical life and all the forms and colors of life, it goes astray. It is the *demand* for things that Christ sets us free from, not things themselves. It is slavery and striving that cease when He comes with His freedom."[13]

The Foundation of Christian Chastity

The word *chastity* is not in the Bible; the word *continence* is not in the

Bible; the words *sexual purity* are not in the Bible. At least, not in the translation offered by the Revised Standard Version, which is the one I am using. So, at first glance, claiming a biblical foundation for a talk about chastity in medical practice would seem difficult indeed. But things are a little different than they appear, because the absence of a word does not necessarily imply the absence of the reality expressed or summarized by that word. To mention an example especially meaningful, one will not find the word *Trinity* in the Bible, either in the Revised Standard Version or in any version, whereas God, One in Three persons, is the foundation of Christian faith.[14] Similarly, even if of much lesser importance, the words *burro* and *donkey* are not in the Bible, but the word *ass*—referring to the same animal—occurs eighty-three times in seventy-three verses. What I mean is that, even if the *word* chastity is not biblical, certainly the *concept* behind that word belongs to the Word of God.

For our purpose it is not necessary to appeal to the Old Testament.[15] Rather, it will suffice to recall one passage from the Gospel and another from the Letters of St. Paul in order to be presented with two fundamental characteristics of chastity in Christian life, and therefore in Christian medical practice.

The first characteristic is its interiority: "out of the heart come evil thoughts, murder, adultery, fornication, theft, false witness, slander."[16] We are faced here with an evangelical perspective that surpasses the previous boundaries of the Mosaic Law: "You have heard that it was said, 'You shall not commit adultery.' But I say to you that every one who looks at a woman lustfully has already committed adultery with her in his heart."[17] In an amazing act of divine authority, Jesus corrects and deepens the old view of adultery. He moves from the level of an external action (with all its obvious characteristics of something public, objective injustice, possibility of scandal, eventual physiological consequences, risk of being stoned to death if caught, etc.) to the level of intention. It is clear that these words of Jesus do not condemn all thoughts about sexual matters; but at the same time it is equally obvious that wishes, desires, looks, imagination, and the like are important in Christian morality.

The second dimension of chastity can be seen in the First Letter to the Corinthians. Man is an incarnated spirit, and this fact influences everything in him, sexuality and human love not excluded. It is obvious that sexual love involves the body; unfortunately, for many people it is not so obvious that the body expresses spiritual love as well. Sex is not something merely biological, like our metabolism or our breathing. It is subject to specific ethical requirements because it is under the influence of our free will and is the expression of something exquisitely human: the capacity to give oneself in love. Only the sexual activities of seriously mentally handicapped people could be exempted from moral implications. As I said, the First Letter to the Corinthians, in its sixth chapter, offers a solid foundation for an interesting reflection. The temptation to reduce the sexual dimension of human beings or their genital activity to an ensemble of physiological mechanisms, anatomical characteristics, hormonal interaction, reflexes of diverse nature, etc., can be very strong. This may be the reason why many people consider medical doctors experts in sexology, even if they don't possess any academic specialization in this field. And this very fact, even if it is not always based on objective reality, adds a new responsibility to the conscience of physicians. We could apply to ourselves some of the sharp questions addressed by St. Paul in the Letter to the Romans: "You then who teach others, will you not teach yourself? . . . You who say that one must not commit adultery, do you commit adultery?"[18] What the First Letter to the Corinthians is emphasizing is that sex cannot be placed at the same level as food or drink. To eat, for example, is only a physiological need and function: "Food is meant for the stomach, and the stomach for food," the Apostle says. "The body is not meant for immorality, but for the Lord, and the Lord for the body."[19] Human sex is not something purely biological. Rather it is deeply related to the intimate Center of the adult human being. In fact, while sexual intercourse seems to be a physical encounter, in reality it expresses the personal and mutual self-giving of a man and a woman, until death. This is why the exercise of human sexuality reaches its true and deepest meaning only in the context of a total, exclusive, and permanent union between a man and a woman (which is the same as saying within marriage).

Sex in Medical Practice

As is well known, the fundamental duties which natural law (or *natural chastity*) imposes on the doctor are considered in the first section of the *Corpus Hippocraticum*, in the famous oath of Hippocrates (born circa 460 BC). One of the duties assumed by those who took the Hippocratic oath was "irreproachable conduct in sexual matters," it being illicit for the doctor to cause repugnance and scandal through illicit familiarity with a patient confided to his care. In the Hippocratic text this precept is extended to perverse sexual activity, with explicit reference to pederasty.

From time to time, we read about physicians who have failed even the test of mere natural decency in their relationships with patients. I don't think that it necessary to recall names and circumstances here and now. More and more, professional bodies and courts of justice are taking care of these sad cases. Somebody could argue that there is no increase in the number of violations of medical ethical code but rather an increase in the publication of these episodes. I am not prepared to contradict this statement. But I suspect that, even if the point were well taken, medical doctors are not immune from the banalization of sex so prevalent in our society. Even more, I am convinced that the fullness of chastity (in medical practice as in any other circumstances of life) cannot be achieved outside the *radiant space* provided by Christian faith; and we have reasons to suspect a tragic absence of genuine Christian life in the perpetuations of such misconduct.

Even if both parties agree to do something evil, evil is still evil. In this context, I invite you to consider again in its totality a passage of the First Letter to the Corinthians, specifically verses 12 and 13 of chapter six: "'All things are lawful for me,' but not all things are helpful. 'All things are lawful for me,' but I will not be enslaved by anything. 'Food is meant for the stomach and the stomach for food'—and God will destroy both one and the other. The body is not meant for immorality, but for the Lord, and the Lord for the body." Many scholars consider today that in this passage St. Paul is giving some answers to false teachings. Let us start with the famous "all things are lawful to me" of verse 12. Is it possible that we are confronted with an immoral Pauline statement? Absolutely not! In fact, this phrase is: a) either a Corinthian slogan,[20] whose application Paul restricts, emphasizing that not everything builds up the community; that some things destroy it;[21] or b) a saying of Paul, which had been perverted at Corinth to justify immorality. In Paul's mouth it meant either "everything not wrong in itself" (i.e., things prohibited in the Jewish ceremonial law, etc.); or "everything which the perfectly spiritual man wishes to do," for he never wishes to do evil and has not thwarted desires.[22]

Let us now apply these ideas to practical results. Medical practice and all that surrounds it can be an occasion for sexual misconduct for a morally weak person. Notice that now I am not talking about things which are specifically banned by a code of ethics; neither am I referring to clamorous cases of scandal, or to types of misdemeanour leading to criminal charges. My main concern aims rather at the inner man, at the specific dimensions of evangelical chastity. In fact I am thinking about ways of talking or looking, which could seem normal and acceptable to the average man or woman, when in fact they are not so before God. I mean lack of consideration for the modesty of the patient, without any specific lecherous intention in the medical staff, but simply because of practicality. In a nutshell, I want to call your attention to everything which could easily pass undetected by current standards and therefore requires a special and attentive effort. I am referring to the indulging in undercover, incomplete acts against chastity, with false exploratory reasons or therapeutic pretences. I am protesting against sexual innuendoes or frivolous comments about the physical characteristics of a patient.

In other words, I am inviting any physician to be "pure in heart"[23] in his or her professional practice, and not only a decent and law abiding citizen, with a clean criminal record. Purity of heart will enable us to see according to God, to accept patients as neighbours in the evangelical sense.[24] With a pure heart we will perceive the human body—ours and our neighbour's—as God's temple,[25] and not only as a biological entity, as a subject for research or as an object for selfish sensual satisfaction.

Wrong Medical Approaches

In medical practice, moral standards should be used to evaluate benefits and burdens. But no positive result can ever justify certain measures. Just to mention an obvious case, it is evident that a possible treatment of a married person's sexual dysfunction by training sessions with another partner is morally wrong in itself and so should be excluded regardless of its prospective benefits.[26]

A particular and controversial case in point is medical intervention in recommending contraception or prescribing drugs, devises or techniques with a contraceptive purpose. I grant that this type of behaviour is socially acceptable; furthermore, it is not easy and fashionable to oppose this trend. But this talk is not about political correctness, but about a deeper understanding of human sexuality, about the divine designs with respect to it and therefore about our personal responsibility in dealing with these issues. We have already considered the two fundamental dimensions of human sexual acts: a) the fact that they are *human* acts, and not merely an epidermic set of sensations or the automatic exercise of a physiological function; b) the fact that human sexual intercourse implies a *mutual self-giving* (unitive aspect) and an *opening to the transmission of life* (procreative aspect).[27]

I do not want to be or to look pessimistic, but it is obvious to me that today's civilization is beset by a profound moral crisis. If we want to search for the reasons, it is important not to forget the impact of a widespread mentality hostile to the sacredness of human life. This hostility shows itself either by suppressing human life when it is no longer wanted (abortion and euthanasia), or manipulating it through the different techniques of human *in vitro* fertilization; or, finally, by avoiding it through the acceptance and practise of artificial contraception.

One may question which comes first, the relaxation of moral norms in general, leading to a contraceptive mentality, or vice versa. Personally I prefer to think, with John Paul II, that at least in the Catholic context, the moral error of refusing to abide by the Church's teaching on contraception has led over the past thirty years to a deeper, wide ranging departure from the basics of Christianity: "The hesitation or doubt of some regarding the moral norm taught by *Humanae vitae* [the document published by Pope Paul VI on family planning on July 25, 1968] has . . . affected other fundamental truths of reason and faith," John Paul II has said.[28]

I offer for your consideration an interesting idea contained in the *Catechism of the Catholic Church*. Probably many of you know already that this *Catechism*, published in October 1992, is the most recent official compendium of Catholic doctrine regarding both faith and morals. In quoting the sixth Beatitude from the Gospel according to Matthew ("Blessed are the pure in heart, for they shall see God"[29]), the *Catechism* states that the pure of heart are those who have surrendered their intelligence and their will to the demands of God's sanctity, mainly in the following three areas: first, charity; second, chastity or sexual rectitude; and third, the love for the truth and the orthodoxy of faith. The reason for the connection between these three areas is specified: there is a link between purity of heart, purity of body, and purity of the faith.[30]

When purity of heart is missing, sound reasoning is weakened, and very easily we end up considering as normal, acceptable, and wonderful what really may be a terrible moral error. "The real history of the world is full of the queerest cases of notions that have turned clean head-over heels and completely contradicted themselves," Chesterton wrote in the early decades of this century. And he specified: "The last example is an extraordinary notion that what is called Birth-Control is a social reform favoured by progressive people. It is rather like saying that cutting off King Charles' head was one of the most elegant of Cavalier fashions in hair dressing. It is like saying that decapitation is an advance on dentistry."[31]

To encourage contraception before marriage means to condone and to foster active sexual life before marriage. It is easy to blame television, modern social trends, or teen irresponsibility. But anybody involved in this problem (and doctors are very much involved) should feel personally touched and challenged. We cannot complain about present cultural misdemeanours, if we don't do what is in our hands to counteract current immoral trends, either before marriage or within it. In this sense, the present contraceptive mentality is a tremendous challenge.

> The innate language that expresses the total reciprocal self-giving of husband and wife is overlaid, through contraception, by an objectively contradictory language, namely, that of not giving oneself totally to the other. This leads not only to a positive refusal to be open to life but also to a falsification of the inner truth of conjugal love, which is called upon to give itself in personal totality.[32]

Somebody could argue that, in not accepting contraception as an option for a patient, the doctor is infringing on the legitimate freedom of this patient; or that he is letting his professional practice be influenced by personal religious convictions. I do not think that this is the case. In the first place, because the goodness or evil of contraception is not a confessional issue, but a human one; it is not a moral or ritual rule commanded by a particular religious denomination, but the consequence of human nature. And in the second place, because a refusal to prescribe contraception can be professionally justified with anthropological, philosophical, and even medical reasons: it is not the easiest way of doing things, but I believe that it is the right one. A doctor cannot be a short-sighted individual, dispensing a remedy for some aspects of life while deeply damaging other interests of the patient in the long run.

I want to finish my talk thanking you for your attention, and telling you that, while I was preparing it and right now, I have being praying that my words may be a vehicle used by the Lord to change our hearts. St. Augustine put it in moving words: "I thought that continence arose from one's own powers, which I did not recognize in myself. I was foolish enough not to know . . . that no one can be continent unless you grant it. For you would surely have granted it if my inner groaning had reached your ears and I with firm faith had cast my cares on you."[33]

Notes

1 Gal 5:16, 19, 21. All scriptural quotations in this article are taken from the Revised Standard Version of the Bible, copyright the Division of Christian Education of the National Council of Churches of Christ in the United States of America.

2 Cf. Rom 3:8. The Catholic tradition, taking as its basis St. Paul's teaching in this passage, has always held that there are some sorts of actions that we must never choose to do, for choosing them is to do evil. St. Augustine expressed this matter vigorously in his Contra Mendacium, c. 7, 18 (PL 40, 528). John Paul II, in his Encyclical The Splendour of Truth has summarized and reinstated this doctrine: "In teaching the existence of intrinsically evil acts, the Church accepts the teaching of Sacred Scripture. The Apostle Paul emphatically states: 'Do not be deceived: neither the immoral, nor idolaters, nor adulterers, nor sexual perverts, nor thieves, nor the greedy, nor drunkards, nor revilers, nor robbers will inherit the Kingdom of God' (1 Cor 6:9-10). If acts are intrinsically evil, a good intention or particular circumstances can diminish their evil, but they cannot remove it. They remain 'irremediably' evil acts; per se and in themselves they are not capable of being ordered to God and to the good of the person" (The

Splendour of the Truth [August 6, 1993], 81).

3 Augustine, *Confessions*, 10, 29, 40: PL 32, 796.

4 Cf. *Catechism of the Catholic Church*, 2522–24

5 Germain Grisez, *The Way of the Lord Jesus*, vol. 2 of *Living a Christian Life* (Quincy, Ill.: Franciscan Press, 1993), 633.

6 Mk 4:22.

7 Mt 6:4, 6, 18.

8 Ex 20:14; Mt 5:27, 19:18; Rom 13:9.

9 1 Jn 4:8, 4:16.

10 Cf. Gal 5:19.

11 Thomas Howard, *Evangelical Is Not Enough* (San Francisco: Ignatius Press, 1984), 32.

12 Gen 1:27-28.

13 Howard, *Evangelical Is Not Enough*, 33.

14 It is generally assumed that the copyright of the word "Trinity" belongs to Tertullian (born circa 155 AD), since he was the first writer to use the Latin word *Trinitas*, as well as *persona*, in the context of Trinitarian theology. There are reasons to believe that Tertullian also introduced the word "chastity" into Christian terminology; a witness to this fact is his *Exhortation to Chastity*. It is addressed to one of his friends who had recently lost his wife. There is no evidence that Tertullian had left the Church when he wrote it; it must thus be dated between 204 and 212 AD (cf. J. Quasten, *Patrology* [Utrecht Antwerp: Spectrum Publishers, 1953], 2:304–5). I must add that the meaning and resonance of the word chastity, as used by Tertullian, has been enormously enriched over eighteen centuries of Christian contemplation and thinking.

15 Cf., to mention only a few examples, Ex 20:14; Lv 20:10; Dt 5:18, 22:20-21, 22:28-29; Prov 6:32; Jer 3:9, 7:9, 23:14.

16 Mt 15:19; cf. also Mk 7:21.

17 Mt 5:27-28.

18 Rom 2:21-22.

19 1 Cor 6:13.

20 Cf. *The New Jerome Biblical Commentary*, ed. R. E. Brown, J. A. Fitzmyer, and R. E. Murphy (Englewood Cliffs, N.J.: Prentice Hall, 1990), 804.

21 Cf. 1 Cor 10:23: "'All things are lawful,' but not all things are helpful. 'All things are lawful,' but not all things build up."

22 Cf. *A Catholic Commentary on Holy Scripture*, gen. ed. B. Orchard (New York: Thomas Nelson & Sons, 1953), 1089.

23 Mt 5:8.

24 Cf. Lk 10:29, 36.

25 Cf. 1 Cor 3:16-17.

26 The reasons for this statement go back to the passage of the Letter to the Ro-

mans already considered in our talk: it is not lawful to "do evil that good may come" (Rom 3:8).

27 On this question it might be useful to consult William E. May, *Sex, Marriage and Chastity: Reflections of a Catholic Layman, Spouse and Parent* (Chicago: Franciscan Herald Press, 1981). In chapter 1, pp. 1–31, Prof. May contrasts the "separatist" understanding of human sexuality widespread in Western societies today with the "integralist" understanding of human sexuality found in the Scriptures and in the Catholic tradition. The separatist understanding, which is predicated on a dualistic understanding of human beings, sees the unitive or amative aspect of human sexuality as the "personal" aspect, while considering the "reproductive" aspect to be something of itself subpersonal and needing to be consciously assumed in order to become human and personal. The integralist understanding, on the other hand, affirms that both the unitive and procreative aspects of our genital sexuality are human and personal. Notice that procreative is not synonymous with reproductive.

28 John Paul II, "Address to the Second International Congress of Moral Theology," November, 12 1988, no. 5, in *Humanae Vitae: 20 anni dopo, Atti del II Congresso Internazionale di Teologia Morale, Roma, November, 9–12, 1988* (Milano: Edizioni Ares, 1989), 16.

29 Mt 5:8.

30 Cf. *Catechism of the Catholic Church*, no. 2518.

31 G. K. Chesterton, "Social Reform versus Birth Control," quoted in *Brave New Family: G. K. Chesterton on Men & Women, Children, Sex, Divorce, Marriage & the Family*, ed. Alvaro de Silva (San Francisco: Ignatius Press, 1990), 193.

32 John Paul II, *Apostolic Exhortation Familiaris Consortio* (November 22, 1981), no. 32.

33 Augustine *Confessions*, 6, 11, 20: PL 32, 729-730.

David Neima

"Evangelium Vitae":
A Physician's Reflections

*E*vangelium vitae was released on March 30, 1995, by Pope John
Paul II. This is the current Pope's eleventh encyclical and follows two years after *Veritatas Splendour*. This document was
assembled over a period of four years with submissions from over
one thousand Bishops from around the world and published after
revision in concert with them. The encyclical is short but very dense
in content with over 142 footnotes. It is a most expressive summary
of a Christian message of life both in the holy scriptures and the
heritage of tradition. This appears to be a singularly useful document to help us meditate on the practice of medicine today from a
positive ethical viewpoint.

The encyclical consists of four main parts. First is a brief introduction which looks at the current attacks on human life. There is a
large second section which focuses on the Christian message of life
which we have in Jesus Christ. The third section is entitled, "God's
Holy Law—you shall not kill," a discussion of the law of God is held
in this section. The final section is entitled, "You did it to me," and
is a call for a new culture of human life to rise from faith in Christ.
The intention of this workshop is to go through all four sections using the scripture quotations as the subsection heads and as the
backbone of the encyclical. Under each heading we will consider the
teaching which is found in the encyclical and apply this to current
medical practice and the ethical questions surrounding it.

Present Day Threats to Human Life
The Incomparable Worth of the Human Person (Lk 2:10-11)
    "I bring you good news of a great joy which will come to

all people, for to you is born this day in the City of
David a Saviour, who is Christ the Lord."[1]
This indeed is the good news of life and the great joy of the birth of
the Saviour and the incarnation of God himself as a small child. He
is the foundation of joy at every child's birth. For Jesus said, "I came
that they may have life, and have it abundantly" (Jn 10:10). Through
the incarnation human life is given an incomparable worth for all
new life and eternal life are the gifts of Jesus. This incarnation principle sets the infinite dignity and value which we must recognize in
every person; the life of every person is an incomparable good which
must ever be set below any thing. We must recognize this gift in each
patient we have, seeing in them a God given dignity. Their lives are
precious treasures for us to guard and never to steal or offend.

Roots of Violence Against Life (Gen 4:8)

"Cain rose up against his brother Abel, and killed him."
The encyclical in effect quotes all of Genesis 4:2-16 which is the first
murder in the world following man's fall in the garden of Eden. To
quote *Evangelium vitae*, "At the root of every act of violence against
one's neighbour, there is the concession to the King of evil, the one
who was a murderer from the beginning" (cf. Jn 8:4).[2] Man's revolt
against God is quickly followed by the deadly combat of man versus
man. We see in the passage quoted that the act of violence is rooted
both in envy and anger and occurs in this case despite God's direct
warning to Abel. There is a deep psychological truth here, that the
roots of anger and envy are present in each person as a result of the
fall. The way of life is also present here as God says to Cain, "You
must master it," (the envy and anger).

As physicians we need to examine our feelings of anger and envy
and we need to question ourselves. Are we angry at our patients? our
colleagues? our government? Are we envious of our patients? co-
workers or colleagues? We must master these feelings, confess them,
and act humbly before our God, realizing our innate feelings and
weaknesses and struggling against them.

Eclipse of the Value of Life (Gen 4:10)

"What have you done?"
This question which God asks Cain is surely put to us today. As phy-

sicians we must regard both our actions and inactions and seek to line them up with God's law and the Gospel. We must keep in mind that the poverty and suffering of millions is indeed at our doorstep, even as Lazarus sat at the doorstep of Dives. In a world of violence, we must be careful to closely examine our practices and conversation to ensure that we do not fall into co-operating with violence to human persons.

Questions to ask ourselves: Do we call people names—"gomers," bad cases, difficult patients? Do we encourage hopelessness by saying that a disease is beyond help, implying that the patient is beyond hope? Do we make a special effort to care for the weak, the poor, and the handicapped, and the dying—or do we avoid these to do easier or more lucrative work? Do we avoid difficult patients? By our silence or inaction do we encourage or allow despair, abortion, or other crimes against life?

A Perverse Idea of Freedom (Gen 4:9)

"Am I my brother's keeper?"
The encyclical lauds society's current movement towards freedom and individual rights, particularly for the individual rights of citizens. On the other hand, it is appalled at the contradictions which unfettered freedom leads to, especially that freedom which is unfettered by truth, which is the love of God. Unfettered, an unnatural freedom leads to crimes against the individual including abortion, euthanasia, and embryo experimentation. An extreme subjectivity with a lack of regard to the absolute truths which God has set on the human person in the world and an exploitation of individual freedom leads to these contradictions. Crimes against the innocent and against the laws of nature result, based on a false freedom. Furthermore, this leads inexorably to an exploitation of the weak. We must remember that freedom is not only individual, but collective. It is expressed in the community and is only true freedom in the context of the truth and God's holy laws. The Christian's answer to the question, "Am I my brother's keeper?" is: "Yes, I am." We are indeed our brother's keepers and this question will be once again asked at the Judgment Day. In particular, as physicians we need to evaluate and question ourselves.

Questions to ask ourselves: Do I make a special effort for patients that other physicians would not like to care for? Do I speak out for the rights of the weak? Do I give time and energy to the elderly, the mentally incompetent, to the very sick or do I finish off with my medical business as quickly as I can? Am I focused on my rights as an earner or on the needs of the sick on my current medical practice? Do I spend more time with the ill and lonely or with the healthy?

The Eclipse of the Sense of God for Man (Gen 4:14)

"And from your face I shall be hidden."

At the heart of violence is the loss of the sense of God. With the loss of the sense of God comes a loss of man's dignity. Life itself becomes a mere thing which man claims as his exclusive property, completely subjected to his control and manipulation. Nature also ceases to be God's good gift to us and events become mere matter for us to use whichever way we choose. From this error comes individualism, materialism, hedonism, and the worse forms of humanism. Values of being are replaced by values of having. So suffering becomes the ultimate evil and religion itself becomes an illness in modern thought. Sexuality becomes depersonalized, exploited, and a mere function as opposed to a sacred gift of God. Personal relationships are grossly impoverished with the loss of the sense of awe for the other. The way back to God is through Christ and the cross.

Questions to ask ourselves as physicians: Do my conversations with patients focus on material ends or on the development of my patients as persons? Do I help them find meaning in suffering? Do I see in each suffering patient the cross of Christ? Do I pray for my patients to know Christ? Do I make a special effort to help the poor by going overseas or by helping here with the disadvantaged? Do I speak of sex and sexual relations with respect and reverence or do I fall into the trap of making it a thing?

Signs of Hope and Invitation to Commitment (Heb 12:22-24)

"You have come to . . . the sprinkled blood."

It is the sprinkled blood of Christ which redeems, purifies, and heals us. This blood which has been shed for all demonstrates how precious is the life of each individual. Due to the shed blood of Christ, we are given the strength to work in hope for the gift of life. Types of work for life that *Evangelium vitae* speaks of include: having children, caring for them, doing good research, volunteering in overseas work, and working to defend the innocent. Surely it also refers to doing good medical practice. In Christ we are indeed part of the culture of life and as physicians must engage actively in conflict with the culture of death.

Questions to ask ourselves: Do I obey God's commandments in my practice? Am I grateful for the salvation in Christ and do I show this in joy and optimism in my counselling and speech to others? Do I support and encourage those who generously have many children? Do I regard each life that I am caring for as worthy of being defended and consecrated to God?

The Christian Life Made Manifest

With Our Gaze Fixed on Christ (1 Jn 1:2)

"The life was made manifest, and we saw it."
We live in a culture which is filled with despair and which crumbles easily in the face of either pain or suffering and the many injustices of modern society. Astonishingly, we are actively discussing the fiduciary worth of various illnesses to determine whether it is worth our while to care for certain persons. Against these contradictions and despair, the gospel of life and Christ stand like a beacon. The assurance of hope and promise of eternal life is present in the person of Christ himself. To be filled with hope and to live this life we need to be rooted firmly in him and in his Gospel. We need to examine ourselves and question ourselves. Do we really believe that Christ is the Lord of life and that there is life eternal? Are we habitually cheerful and pleasant?

Life Is Always Good (Ex 15:2)

"The Lord is my strength and my song, and he has become my salvation."
The encyclical looks at the scriptural examples of hope under the motifs of the suffering of the nation of Israel under Egypt, of Job in severe illness, and the person of Christ suffering for us his passion on the cross. To note the words of *Evangelium vitae* section 31, "truly great must be the value of human life, if the Son of God has taken it up and made it the instrument of the salvation of humanity."

Throughout salvation history in the Old and New Testaments, life is always regarded as a good. The example we are set in all sorts of suffering, in bondage and captivity, is to look to God and place our hope and trust in him. There may indeed seem to be no earthly hope but life is truly good because it is a gift from God and there is always an eternal hope in him attached to it.

Questions we need to ask ourselves: As physicians do we give up on hopeless cases? Do we get tired of the patient we see over and over again with the same complaint? Do we find despair in our hearts and allow it to be communicated to our patients? Do we find faith in Christ and communicate this through optimism and hope and even through his name when the opportunity presents itself?

Jesus Brings Life's Meaning to Fulfilment (Acts 3:16)

"His name . . . has made this man strong."
Peter cured the cripple at the Beautiful gate in the name of Jesus. In truth, all healing comes from him. In addition, much of our malaise is from sin and a lack of recognition of the innate value of each person. Only an encounter with Jesus can give the full authenticity of life to the lost and the suffering. As physicians we must be prudent and honest, practising our skills to the best of our ability and recognizing our own limitations. At the same time we have a great advantage as Christians and should recognize that much parades as illness which can only be cured today, in fact, by the name of Jesus.

Questions to ask ourselves: Do we frankly let patients know when we think that their problems are not medical? In our conversations with the ill or with patients with spiritual problems does the name of God ever appear? While we should not push our faith, we should not be hiding it and the name of the Lord should be natural to our conversation.

God's Glory Shines in the Face of Man (Rom 8:28-29)

"Called . . . to be conformed to the image of his Son."
Evangelium vitae reminds us once again that we are formed in the image of God and therefore of infinite value. Due to the fall, this image is tarnished and subjected to sickness, sin and death. But it has been restored in Christ. "The first man Adam became a living being; the last Adam became a life-giving spirit" (1 Cor 15:45). We

are called to the restoration of life in the image of the Son. This call is both to us individually and to action as regards others. We are called to restore the sick and the lame and to give hope where it is lost. This is our call and it can be seen as our duty to try to help others both to health and to growth in the *imago Dei*—that is, through the Gospel.

Question for ourselves as physicians: Do we see our primary tasks as healers to help others to conform to the wonderful image of Christ in God?

The Gift of Eternal Life (Jn 11:26)

"Whoever lives and believes in me shall never die."

In Jesus we have already begun an everlasting life. We need to recognize, therefore, that death is not the end point of this life but rather the potential gate to eternal life which alone is this life's true goal. How then can we as those who dwell and live for eternal life dispense death through euthanasia or abortion or frustrate life through acts of contraception? Eternal life should make us intensely aware that each human life is not given its meaning by its condition on earth but by its eternal destination. It is neither health, intelligence, strength, or wealth but life eternal in Christ which counts and makes each person valuable. So children, the elderly, the severely ill and mentally handicapped are not truly bound by their weaknesses but in truth by their relationship to Christ.

We must recognize that every life is worthy of our care and dedication. We should have a confidence and joy in caring for the unfortunate that will lead others to question how we are able to bear up. We must take this opportunity to tell them about him who is the resurrection and the life.

Reverence and Love for Every Human Life (Gen 9:5)

"From man in regard to his fellow man I will demand
an accounting" (NAB).

From the ten commandments we learn, "You shall not kill" (Ex 20:13), which is the true moral absolute. We cannot do as we will with the lives of ourselves or others. For this, we are accountable to God. Our Lord Jesus expands accountability to include even anger in Matthew 5:21-22. Also, in the parable of the good Samaritan we learn that responsibility does indeed extend to strangers for whom we are also accountable (Lk 10:25-37).

As a physician I conclude that we must reverence and serve human lives, even those of our enemies. These lead to questions to ask ourselves: Am I reluctant or do I refuse to care for patients who are threatening or disturbing? Do I avoid caring for those who do not appreciate my work? Do I make as much effort to care for the disgruntled as well as the pleasant patient?

Man's Responsibility for Life (Gen 1:28)

"Be fruitful and multiply and fill the earth and subdue it."
Through his command, we share in God's dominion over the earth. We especially share in his dominion through our fertility. Eve exclaims, "I have gotten a man with the help of the Lord" (Gen 4:1). Every child is a creation of God through the co-operation of the spouses. This means that God transmits his image to the new creature, the child; and so parents are led to responsibility for the education and nurturing of this new life. Christ added to this natural responsibility, responsibility for the sick, the naked, and the prisoner (Mt 25:31-46).

Questions to ask ourselves: Do we as physicians recognize the presence of God in the act of procreation? Do we speak of this subject and treat it with the reverence which is due to the presence of our Lord? Do we help others realize how wonderful and extraordinary this physical action is? Do we speak of it with the tact and delicacy necessary to respect the spouse's and God's rights?

The Dignity of the Unborn Child (Ps 139:13)

"For thou didst form my inward parts."
The life of every individual from its very beginning is a part of God's plan, "Before I formed you in the womb, I knew you, and before you were born I consecrated you" (Jer 1:5). In the discussion in *Evangelium vitae*, the writers point out that direct calls to protect the life of the unborn child are not found in the Old Testament due to the enormous value given to new life. "Sons are a heritage from the Lord, the fruit of the womb a reward" (Ps 127:3). A quote from St. Ambrose regarding the visitation points out that John the Baptist was sanctified in his mother's womb and so being sanctified, sancti-

fied and inspired his mother Elizabeth. This sanctification came from the unborn child Jesus in the womb of his mother Mary—great respect and honour is given to these unborn children in the gospel account we find in Luke.

We must be careful always to recognize the dignity of the unborn child, one which is given by God and exemplified by Jesus and John the Baptist in their mother's wombs. When dealing with a pregnancy, do we always talk of *the baby* and consider the dignity and wonder of the unborn child? Do we rejoice at the discovery of a pregnancy, regardless of the situation, rejoicing at God's infinite gift?

Life in Old Age and at Times of Suffering (Ps 116:10)
"I kept my faith, even when I said, 'I am greatly afflicted.'"
Even in pain and suffering we are to continue to hope in God. Life may be surrendered, as Stephen did, and as our Lord did on the cross, but it must not be taken. Jesus sends his disciples out to heal (Mt 10:7-8). Similarly, we are sent out as physicians to heal and do good. We need to trust in God and to help our patients trust, especially if they are greatly afflicted. If our patients lack faith, we must not lack ours as well but hold fast and encourage the suffering patient. As Christians we must not regard suffering as either meaningless or as punishment, but must through the cross see its redemptive value. This should in no way hinder our attempts to relieve suffering, but focus our compassion and prayer for the suffering patient.

From the Law of Sinai to the Gift of the Spirit (Bar 4:1)
"All who hold her fast will live."
Evangelium vitae section 48 states, "Life is indelibly marked by a truth of its own." The laws of the covenant including, "Thou shall not kill" (Ex 20:13) are truths which undergird life's absolute morals without which no ethic or morality can hold. Without these truths, so called morality departs from truth and therefore from freedom. In Jesus we see the fulfilment of the law and its transformation to "the law of the Spirit of life in Christ Jesus" (Rom 8:2), which is the law of love. It must be emphasised that this law in no way contradicts the ten commandments or is in conflict with them. It is a simple absurdity to claim that the law of love can override any of the ten commandments or be contrary to any natural morality. Love is a call

to a higher morality and not a lower one. We may surrender ourselves in love to God through our work for our brothers and sisters. This is the law of life. It is ourselves who are surrendered and not the law of God, of which Jesus said that not one jot or tittle would pass away before the passing of this world.

A question to ask ourselves in this regard is whether we love our patients in this way, ready to surrender our rights but never God's laws?

The Gospel of Life Is Brought to Fulfilment on the Tree of the Cross (Jn 19:37)
"They shall look on him whom they have pierced."
The central message of our faith is found on the cross at Calvary. Here in the death of Jesus, and through his total self sacrifice for us, we find new life. Through his suffering and death we find meaning and hope in ours. The cross can lead us to praise even amidst the despair of dark, suffering, and death. Through the darkness of the Good Fridays of our lives, and the lives of others, the life of the resurrection of Easter Sunday should shine.

Questions to ask ourselves: Are we silent when patients speak about their own death, or the deaths of those loved by them? Do we share a confidence in the resurrection and in life after death? Do we pray for those who are dying and for those who have died?

God's Holy Law
Gospel and Commandment (Mt 19:17)
"If you would enter life, keep the commandments"
Evangelium vitae examines, as does *Veritatas Splendour*, the event of the rich young ruler who approaches Jesus. In Jesus' reply to the rich young ruler we see that God's commandment is never detached from his Life, nor from life. Similarly, our care as physicians should never be detached, either from the love of God or his commandments. The gift of the gospel and of new life in Christ becomes for us a commandment to do good. Ethical freedom and true morality are founded within the law of God. Commandments can be likened to the solid ground in which we walk in true freedom, for there is no true freedom apart from truth and indeed God's law is the truth.

A question to ask ourselves: Do we always remember that no

good can come to our patients through the breaking of the least of God's laws?

Human Life is Sacred and Inviolable (Gen 9:5)
"From man in regard to his fellow man, I will demand an accounting for human life" (NAB).
God alone is the Lord of life from its beginning until its end. No one can in any circumstance claim for himself the right to destroy directly an innocent human being.[3] The Didache teaches, "There are two ways, a way of life and a way of death."[4] Didache goes on to condemn abortions and failure to help the sick. This was written in the first century and shows the continuing tradition of the protection of life and care for the sick which was found amongst the earliest Christians and continues to be the core of Christian witness to the sanctity of life and the gift of new life which we have in Christ. Only legitimate self defence, and this only to the amount needed to defend life, is permitted. In *Evangelium vitae* the question is raised whether there is any place in modern society for the death penalty. Section 52 of *Evangelium vitae* states, "I confirm that the direct and voluntary killing of an innocent human being is always gravely immoral." Shortly thereafter it states, "Every innocent human being is absolutely equal to all others." This statement is the formation of the basics of true justice and one to which we as physicians must absolutely adhere.

We must question ourselves: Do we ever make the mistake of valuing one human life above that of another in our treatment? Do we in any way contribute to the death of the innocent either by acts of co-operation or acts of omission?

The Unspeakable Crime of Abortion (Ps 139:16)
"Thy eyes beheld my unformed substance."
Our society's acceptance of abortion is a moral crisis. We must be careful as Christian physicians to call things by their proper names. "Woe to those who call evil good and good evil, who put darkness for light and light for darkness" (Is 5:20). We must be very clear in our speech about what abortion is—the deliberate killing of an innocent human being. Both in language and in action there is a network of societal complicity in our high abortion rates. *Evangelium*

vitae section 59 states, "We are facing what can be called a structure of sin which opposes human life not yet born. A human being is to be respected and treated as a person from the moment of conception." Likewise, *Evangelium vitae* condemns experimentation on embryos which is not for their direct benefit.

We must question ourselves whether we in our speech fail to clear the atmosphere around the abortion debate. Do we in any way contribute in our medical practice to the structure of sin that promotes abortion? Are we actively providing the support that women need to take care of children, to have their babies and not kill them?

The Tragedy of Euthanasia (Dt 32:39)

"It is I who bring both death and life" (NAB).

In *Evangelium vitae* section 64 we read, "Euthanasia's terms of reference, therefore, are to be found in the intention of the will and in the methods used . . . one can in conscience refuse forms of treatment that would only secure a precarious and burdensome prolongation of life, so long as the normal care due to the sick person in similar cases is not interrupted." This is the principle of double effect where pain killers, for example, and palliative care is strongly encouraged by *Evangelium vitae*. The deliberate ending of life, however, is clearly forbidden. *Evangelium vitae* section 86 states that, "Suicide is always as morally objectionable as murder." Further, we read, "true compassion leads to sharing another's pain: it does not kill the person whose suffering we cannot bear." *Evangelium vitae* section 67 says, "Yet it (a suicide request), is a plea for help to keep on hoping when all human hope fails."

We must indeed always seek to relieve suffering but never play God. The beginning and end of life are clearly in God's hands and should never be in our ours.

Civil Law and Moral Law (Acts 5:29)

"We must obey God rather than men."

Our present day culture is carefully devised by marked ethical relativism. A democratic majority has decided that abortion should be legal, which has led to a terrible tyranny, the slaughter of the innocent. We must remember that democracy is a system, a means, and not an end and can in no way substitute for the truth. Through democratic means we must struggle for the truth and we must never accept the majority's will as truth. This simple distinction seems to be lost on modern culture. Civil law should not remove or replace moral laws but rather obey them, especially the natural law which forbids the taking of innocent life. *Evangelium vitae* section 72 states, "When the law is contrary to reason it is called an unjust law. In this case it ceases to be a law and becomes instead an act of violence." *Evangelium vitae* section 73, "There is a grave and clear obligation to oppose them (abortion and euthanasia) by conscientious objection." The example of the Hebrew midwives is given to encourage and not to co-operate in the killing of the innocent. Legislative voters, it is noted, may choose the least evil option, always seeking and arguing towards the truth.

We must examine closely our medical practices to see if we in any way co-operate with the death of the innocent. Are we active through democratic means in our struggle to promote the truth and to move our culture towards the culture of life?

Promote Life (Lk 10:27)
"You shall love . . . your neighbour as yourself."
"You shall not kill" is a law that is the lower limit of Christian behaviour. This precept should be the start of the promotion of life. We are truly entrusted to one another as a reflection of the mutual self-giving of the most Holy Trinity.

For our reflection: Do I see myself as caring for my neighbour in my medical practice? Does my profession actively promote and care for human life? Are there problems in my community that I should be addressing through my medical practice? Am I taking the time required to truly care for each one of my patients? Do I measure my care in medicine by the standard of love, which is Christ's banner, or do I look at material values only?

You Did It to Me—For a New Culture of Human Life
A People of Life and for Life (1 Pet 2:9)
"You are . . . God's own people, that you may declare the wonderful deeds of him who called you out of darkness into his magnificent life."
Evangelium vitae illustrates that the call to evangelize which is given

to each Christian is also a call to spread the message of life. We are sent by our Lord and as physicians we must especially serve life, seeking to develop programs and structures which promote life. We are sent furthermore as a people and therefore must work together as a Christian community to call our society back to respect the sanctity of life. In justice it is our moral duty to preach the message of life through our practice, in our conversation, and in our prayer.

Proclaiming the Gospel of Life (1 Jn 1:3)
> "That which we have seen and heard we proclaim also
> to you."

Jesus himself is the Gospel. We must not allow our medical practice to be separated from him. How can it be that the servants of life work, except under the Lord of life himself? He must be in our minds as we practise, in our hands as we labour, and with naturalness and ease on our lips when the occasion arises. Our faith and medical practice should and must be one, or our medical practice will soon become a part of the culture of death. This means that we must have both professional excellence and maintain the presence of God while we are working. We must remember that we are called to be physicians and not preachers, but that our work must always be performed unto the Lord.

Celebrating the Gospel of Light (Ps 139:14)
> "I give you thanks that I am fearfully, wonderfully
> made" (NAB).

The person of each individual is a great wonder and a tremendous gift. We need to have a contemplative outlook in order to celebrate the Gospel of life seeing each individual as God's creation. We must remember that life is a gift and not a possession. We must treat our patients thanking God for their life. Through an act of contemplation and faith in God, we will be able to see beauty in every life and in every patient that we treat. *Evangelium vitae* points out that we must use the wealth of mysteries and symbols in every culture to celebrate life. This will include for the physician a real effort to learn about our patients' traditions and celebrations in their varying cultures with a real effort to accept and help what is noble in these. We should make a gift of ourselves to others as physicians and help those who are making gifts of themselves, especially mothers who care and suffer for their children.

Questions to ask ourselves: As doctors do we pray for our patients and thank God for the life of each one? Do we take the time to celebrate life with them, their births, marriages, deaths, and special seasons of worship, even if not Christian?

Serving the Gospel of Life (Jas 2:14)

> "What does it profit, my brethren, if a man says he has faith but has not works?"

The gospel of life calls us to charity and to active service according to our ability. There is in particular a need for doctors to speak and to be actively serving life in the face of this culture of death. We should indeed have a preference and service for the poor, the truly sick, and the neglected of this world. We should be careful to care for those that our colleagues prefer not to care for. *Evangelium vitae* section 87 says, "We must care for the other as a person for whom God has made us responsible." We must also educate our colleagues about the gift of life and the joy that we have through this gift in God. A real commitment to life and self giving in marriage, to the value of children and the sanctity of sexuality should shine throughout our medical practices. We must be committed to care for the dying, especially those for whom euthanasia may be an attraction.

The Family Is the Sanctuary of Life" (Ps 128:3)

> "Your children will be like olive shoots around your table."

As physicians we must be especially careful to be responsible to our families. This includes receiving the children which God gives us and giving them the time and nurturing which they need. We must structure our work around our children's true needs. The family should be the sanctuary of life, a domestic church. Daily prayer in our families is needed and consideration to adoption and helping our children's friends should be given as well. A truly Christian medical practice is founded on a Christian home. A Christian medical practice will flounder on a family neglected for the "higher calling" of medicine. Such a misconception can only lead to mistreatment of patients as well. How can we love our patients if we do not first love our spouses and children? How can we love medicine if we do not take the time to pray and worship God? The hierarchy of God, life, family, and work must be diligently attended to by physicians or their patients will indeed pay the price for their doctor's disordered life.

Bringing About the Transformation of Culture (Eph 5:8-11)
> "Walk as children of light . . . and try to learn what is pleasing to the Lord. Take no part in the unfruitful works of darkness."

As physicians we especially need to be transformed interiorly and to walk continually in his presence. We also need to study, as the text points out, and learn what is pleasing to our Lord in our profession, both by technical excellence and moral excellence. We should be participating in conferences on medical ethics and it is our duty to learn what is pleasing to the Lord in our work, both ecclesiastically and through professional competence. We must also actively avoid doing those things which do not please the Lord, even if we are taught them in medical school or if they are lawful, convenient, or even required. It is right that we should be actively Christian doctors amongst our fellow churchgoers and parishioners, discussing the rights and wrongs of medicine with them and speaking out as well in our medical societies. We need to be diligent in forming our own consciences and help others to recover the necessary link between truth and freedom. We need also to speak of the meaning of healthy sexuality. It is also necessary to speak openly about suffering and death and its meaning through the cross of Christ. The primacy of people over things must be central in our speech. It is popular today to attack the sick as drains on society and as physicians we ought to be advocates for them and for the acceptance and care of children, the unborn, the elderly, and dying. We should help pregnant women to accept their children with joy and those who have had abortions to find forgiveness and new life in Christ.

The Gospel of Life is for the Whole of Human Society (1 Jn 1:4)
> "We are writing this that our joy may be complete."

It is important to note that the gospel of life is for all and not just for believers. Because this gospel is founded on Jesus Christ it is universal and not limited to ourselves. In conversation with all patients, not just Christians, we should naturally share our reverence for their person and for the sanctity of their lives. Life is a gift, let us thank God for that gift in the face of suffering, remembering in our hearts how Our Lord suffered for us.

The Motherhood of Mary and of the Church (Rev 12:1)
> "A great portent appeared in heaven, a woman clothed
> with the sun."

The church is the seed of the kingdom of God and its beginning on earth. As did Mary, the church bears within herself the saviour of the world, Christ our Lord. In Mary we see the new Eve raising earthly motherhood to its highest vocation. The church today, like Mary, has to live its motherhood in suffering. Even as Mary stood by Jesus on the cross, we too must stand beside those who are suffering and dying. Like Mary we should bear their sufferings within ourselves. As John did at the foot of the cross, it is wise for us also to take Mary as our mother. When we are with the sick and dying, let us enter spiritually and interiorly into that special family at Calvary.

Life Menaced by the Forces of Evil (Rev 12:4)
> "And the dragon stood before the woman . . . that he
> might devour her child when she brought it forth."

Even so Mary and Joseph had to flee into Egypt to protect Jesus. How many children today die devoured by the devil and evil sewn in the hearts of men and women! In Mary and Jesus we see every child who is threatened, every unborn baby—for to all of these innocents Christ has united himself. Rejection of human life is truly a rejection of Christ. "Whoever receives one such child in my name, receives me" (Mt 18:5). "Truly, I say to you, as you did it to one of these the least of my brethren, you did it to me" (Mt 25:40). We must help save the lives of our innocents today, we must as real doctors struggle against our modern day Herods. May we be as chaste as Joseph, with every patient of the opposite sex.

The Splendour of the Resurrection (Rev 21:4)
> "Death shall be no more."

When Gabriel announced the conception of Jesus to Mary he said,

"Do not be afraid, Mary" and "with God nothing shall be impossible" (Lk 1:30, 37). The whole of Mary's life is pervaded with the presence of God, even though it is filled with struggles and contradictions and includes the death of her only Son. But Jesus is risen and in truth death shall be no more. We too should take the advice that Gabriel gave to Mary and "be not afraid." We should care for each of our patients as she cared for Jesus, confident in him that death will be destroyed. As she stood at the foot of the cross, Mary's heart was pierced by the sword of compassion, even as Simeon had prophesied. We too must be ready to open our hearts to the suffering of the sick and innocent.

Notes

[1] Unless otherwise noted, all scriptural quotations in this article are taken from the Revised Standard Version of the Bible, copyright the Division of Christian Education of the National Council of Churches of Christ in the United States of America.

[2] Pope John Paul II, *Evangelium vitae*, Encyclical Letter, (Boston: Pauline Books and Media, 1995).

[3] Catechism of the Catholic Church, no. 2258.

[4] *Didache* 1.1, *Patres Apostlici*, ed. F. X. Funk.

Part II

Virtue of Hope

Edwin C. Hui

Hope, Stewardship, and Medical Technology

O
f the four recurring human puzzlements and agonies—
death, suffering, sin, and ignorance—which people of all
times, cultures, and religions have to confront and to cope,[1]
the medical profession has traditionally been called to engage people
under the grips of suffering. On the surface, it may appear that it is
the skills of the practitioner and the responsiveness of the patient
that provide relief to the patient; but beneath the surface, it is ultimately "hope" that neutralizes the sting of people's suffering. Every
medical intervention, whether it be preventive, interventive, palliative, or otherwise, is mediated by hope, both on the part of the patient as well as the provider; we seek and provide intervention because we hope that "what is" can be made into "what should be."
Sometimes we succeed, sometimes we don't. But the grip of suffering is loosened because the hope affirms that the patient's suffering
matters and that there is meaning to the condition of the patient.
Hope symbolizes meaning and removes the pain and suffering. In
this sense, hope is not an objective estimation of a particular situation or a prognostication of a condition. Vaclav Havel, the brilliant
Czech president, put it well when he said that "[hope] is not the
conviction that something will turn out well, but the certainty that
something makes sense, regardless of how it turns out."[2] Today, people in different parts of the world are crying for release from the
grips of suffering of one kind or the other, and the antidote is rightly
hope as Desmond Tutu captured well in his book title as well as in
his life: *Hope and Suffering*.[3] The cry for release from suffering and
the quest for hope are the preoccupation of our time. The first task
of this essay is to review the theological virtue of hope and see how it

functions in the Christian life. The second task is to show how the loss of genuine hope has led to a specific suffering of modernity: the tyranny of unchecked and limitless development of technology. And the third task is to remind ourselves that the Christian character of accountable stewardship shaped by our hope in God is the only proper guide for the development and application of medical technology.

Definition of Hope

It is not easy to define hope because it is both a diffuse and inclusive concept. We may try to describe hope under two categories, psychological and ontological.

Psychological Structure of Hope

Subjectively in the human psyche, hope is an expectant attitude which involves cognitive, emotional, volitional, as well as spiritual dimensions. It is rooted in one's desire and trust. The desire which leads to hope is a way one approaches life in expectation of some future goals, future-oriented actions, future objects, or to borrow G. Fackre's phrase: "a trajectory into the future." Without this concrete external object of expectation, hope remains a wish, which is a counterfeit of hope. Subjectively, hope as an attitude also consists of trust or confidence which in turn may be grounded in either some supernatural or metaphysical forces, or in natural forces which are one's ability to achieve the objective in view. Desire and confidence are related because a hopeful desire has credibility only when there is confidence that it is achievable, or at least a minimal degree of probability that it can be accomplished. Hope without a measure of confidence or trust about the future object hoped for is a shallow optimism, which is another counterfeit of hope.[4] The more daring and imaginative the hope, the greatest the trust one must have in the future. For example, some social reformers or political activists may entertain a hope which embraces a whole nation or even the entire human race. At this level, there may be a danger that the confidence or trust one has in the future is so removed from reality that the hope is merely a form of utopianism. Such hope is a mere illusion, a third counterfeit of hope.

Because of the importance of hope in the human psyche, psychologists have emphasized its importance in three areas. In the first place, hope is important in human motivation. Psychiatrist A. T. Beck observed that hopelessness is the dominant feature of all mod-erate to severe depressive patients and is present in 50% of the milder cases of depression. He concludes that "Hopelessness is at the top of the list of cognitive patterns that underlie depression."[5] Secondly, hope has an important role in human personality. Contemporary personality theorists emphasize the significance of "purpose" as the most creative force in the development of human personality. In their absence, significant distortion in personality can be expected. And finally, medical practitioners have long affirmed the curative power of hope. Timothy R. Elliott, a counselling psychologist, studied patients with spinal cord injuries and found that those with hope who continued to have a purpose in their lives recovered better than those who didn't.[6] Another research team, M. F. Scheier and C. S. Carver, discovered that middle-aged men recovering from heart bypass surgery had a faster rate of physical healing as reflected in their quicker hospital discharge rate and earlier return to work and normal activities if their disposition was the hopeful type.[7] The medical literature is filled with these examples. The prevalence of hope in human personality and behaviour raises the question whether or not hope can be viewed as part of the human nature.

Ontological Structure of Hope

At first sight, hope is a concept so elusive that it may not be counted on to provide a firm datum for a philosophy of human nature, and even less for a general philosophy with metaphysical or ontological significance. Yet two prominent philosophers of this century have written about hope as if it is quite central to human nature and existence.

The first one is Ernst Bloch, a neo-Marxist who wrote his three-volume magnum opus *Principle of Hope* in which he sees the human being in a process of transcendence and it is hope that draws him on to new levels of being. He says, "The human being has still much in front of him. He is constantly being transformed in and through his work. He is constantly standing before boundaries which cease to be such as he perceives and surpasses them. What is authentic in humanity as in the world waits in its potentiality, fearing frustration and hoping for success."[8] By referring to both the human being and the world, Bloch is claiming that hope is a potentiality characteristic not only of the human race but the whole universe as well. For this reason, in Bloch's philosophy, hope is not just a human or sociological principle but in some sense also a metaphysical principle. Even though Bloch remained an atheist all his life, he himself was doubtful whether such a metaphysic of hope or a "total hope" for the human race and the universe can be sustained without some religious interpretation. In his own words, he said, "Where there is hope, there is religion."[9]

The second philosopher who has spoken explicitly of a "metaphysic of hope" is Gabriel Marcel who belongs to a tradition very different from Bloch's. Like Bloch, Marcel thought of the human being as in a process of transcendence; man is, in Marcel's own expression (which also serves as the title of his book), *homo viator*, on his way towards a fuller and more authentic humanity. But unlike Bloch who conceived the goal of the human journey to be more or less self-made and self-chosen, Marcel was a theist and believed that the end of the human transcendence is participation in the transcendent being of God. Marcel did not construct his metaphysic of hope on abstract speculation, but rather on a phenomenology of the human condition which he claimed to reveal that hope is virtually omnipresent in everything we do. Marcel notes the simplest and even trivial hopes, hopes "of a low order" that enter into one's everyday life and argues that they are precursors to larger hopes. In his view, trivial hopes imply other hopes which in turn allows us to see the world in a hopeful way. Such a predisposition also implies a ground of hope beyond the human act of hoping and it is this, according to Marcel, that differentiates hope from optimism which is only a matter of the human ego. Indeed, if hope is the spur to transcendence and if hope also implies trust in the future, then the very presence of hope in the world is highly suggestive of and even demands an ultimate transcendent ground of hope, i.e., a belief in a God with a fully eschatological theology. It is interesting in this regard that Vaclav Havel, despite his lack of a religious belief, nevertheless recognizes that hope's "deepest roots are in the transcendental . . . ." This is what he says of hope: "It is a dimension of the soul, . . . an orientation of the Spirit, an orientation of the heart; it transcends the world that is immediately experienced, and is anchored somewhere beyond its horizons."[10] And in the Judeo-Christian tradition, such a hope from beyond has revealed himself as the God of Israel.

The Jewish Tradition of Hope

There are three main contributions Judaism has made to the idea of God, and they all have something to do with hope.[11]

First, the idea that there is one God, Jehovah (Yahweh), who is unlike any other God and totally different from humankind. He is transcendent, all powerful, all knowing, and totally righteous. He is uniquely and absolutely one. Yet secondly, the Jews believe, as Christians do, that at the same time this just and Holy One God is a personal God. The revolutionary contribution of Judaism is its utter radical idea of the character of God: transcendent and infinite, yet personal, revealing his heart to humankind, stern against immorality and disobedience, yet merciful to those who repent and moved to action by our sufferings and petitions—a living and personal God to whom people can come with their longings, love, tears, praises, fears, and hopes. The third contribution is universalism in Judaism. Judaism asserts that Yahweh is not only God of the Jews but the God of all nations. God's calling upon the Jews is part of his larger plan to bring all nations under his sovereignty. Yahweh specifically told Abram that "all peoples on earth will be blessed through you" (Gen 12:3)[12] and he repeats the promise to Isaac that "through your offspring all nations on earth will be blessed" (Gen 26:4). This is a revelation of the divine will for the whole human race, a revelation which was rooted in the historical events of the Jewish part, yet at the same time lays claim to the unfolding of future history. The greatest source of confidence in the Jewish tradition is not so much that God has revealed a set of moral precepts or that he has promised them blessings, but rather the conviction that God has disclosed his plans for the human race and he will remain in charge of history until the very end of time.

Milton Steinberg summarizes the Jewish tradition of hope in what he calls "the triple hope" of Judaism:

1. The expectation of ultimate deliverance and vindication

2. The hope of the survival of the individual soul

3. The hope of regeneration of the society[13]

The triple hope is the concept of God's Kingdom, which the Jews have believed would literally be inaugurated by the Messiah. For this reason, the Jewish vision of God's kingdom is often called the Messianic hope.

Hope in the Old Testament

The English word hope occurs at least ninety-five times in the New International Version of Old Testament translating four different yet closely related Hebrew words: tiqwah, yahal, qawahl, and miqwehl. Tiqwah is translated to "hope" more than any other Hebrew word in the Bible. In its Hebrew form, tiqwah is concrete and positive. Zophar assures Job "You will be secure, because there is hope [tiqwah]; you will look about you and take your rest in safety" (Job 11:18). In the Old Testament, everybody is said to possess hope. The poor have hope (Job 5:16), the afflicted have it (Ps 9:18), and even the wicked have hope (Prov 11:23). This is so because the Hebrew people know that hope comes from God himself who does not discriminate (Ps 62:5, 71:5; Prov 23:18). God alone is the source of tiqwah.

The verb yahal connotes an utter dependence and confidence, a confidence that is quite independent of the situation. The most dramatic use was by Job when he said "Though he slay me, yet will I hope [yahal] in him" (Job 13:15). Its usage has an implicit trusting relationship with the person in whom hope is put. The one looked to is God, and the context is always an expectation that he will respond (Ps 33:22; 42:5; 42:11; 43:5; 119:43, 49, 74, 81, 114).

Qawahl differs from yahal in that it connotes of future time. In twelve cases, qawahl is translated as "wait" or "wait for" referring to God and in expectation that God will be involved. In Psalm 40:1 "I waited patiently for the Lord; he turned to me and heard my cry."

Miqwehl occurs only five times in the Old Testament and yet on each occasion it is translated as hope. It is the prophet Jeremiah who makes it clear that this special word has a special and important meaning that the other words do not have because the word is nothing less than God himself. In a prayer of great distress when God is about to punish the unfaithful Judah, Jeremiah implores: "O Hope of Israel, its Saviour in times of distress, why are you like a stranger in the land, like a traveler who stays only a night?" (Jer 14:8). In essence, *miqwehl* is the collective hope of the Jewish people, the personal Almighty God himself.

New Testament Hope

It is fair to say that the central theme of Jesus' message is hope. The good news of the gospel is not just about the wrath of God and the forgiveness of sin, it is about a new future, or a new creation which God has prepared for men. The link between the present man and the new man of the future is "the glorious riches of this mystery, which is Christ in you, the hope of glory" (Col 1:27). Paul was persecuted because he offered this gospel hope which is based on a new relationship with God through the Messiah. In Caesarea, he explained to King Agrippa and Queen Bernice: "It is because of my hope in what God has promised our fathers that I am on trial today" (Acts 26:6). And in Rome, he said the same thing to the Jewish leaders: "It is because of the hope of Israel that I am bound with this chain" (Acts 28:20).

The primary hope of the gospel is the identification of the Messianic promise of the Old Testament with Jesus of Nazareth. As the author of Hebrews explains, the Law—the old covenant—simply was not capable of making men and women morally perfect. There was the need for another priest to come, "one in the order of Melchizedek" (Heb 7:11); and there is the need for a better hope, by which we draw near to God (Heb 7:18-19). The "better hope" is simply access for all believers in Jesus to the "Most Holy Place." And that access is gained through the one-time sacrifice of Jesus. This incredible access to God's mercy and grace is "the hope we profess" which we must "hold unswervingly to" (Heb 10:23) as "an anchor for the soul, firm and secure" (Heb 6:19), the very foundation of Christian life.

There are four aspects under which we need to understand the distinctive features of New Testament hope: its content, its basis, its nature, and its purpose.

The Content of New Testament Hope Is Christ

Christ himself is called the Christian hope (1 Tim 1:1), and by his resurrection the virtue of Christian hope is bestowed on the believer through the Spirit (Rom 15:13). Perhaps the best statement testifying to the Christocentricity of the New Testament hope is the fact that the word hope (*elpis*) does not appear even once in the last book of the Bible. This is because the resurrected Christ, in his appearance to John in the vision on the Isle of Patmos, is himself present as the speaker in the Book of Revelation. Hope was almost absent from the Gospels for the same reason. Jesus Christ, the *Alpha* and the *Omega*, is present in Revelation and the Gospels. And so it seems more appropriate that the last words of Revelation and indeed the whole of Scripture, brings together the Messianic hope, the Messiah, and God's kingdom by the ultimate cry of hope: "Amen. Come, Lord Jesus." (Rev 22:20); for in John's eyes, the Lord Jesus is Luke's "hope of Israel" (Acts 28:20), Peter's "living hope" (1 Pet 1:3), and Paul's "God of hope" (Rom 15:13), who is also simply and powerfully "our hope" (1 Tim 1:1-2). The heart of hope is not the blessing of the individual but the universal kingly rule of God, in which he will be "all in all." Its object is the ultimate blessedness of God's Kingdom (Acts 2:2; Tit 1:2). Its content is therefore defined as salvation (1 Thess 5:8) and includes the resurrection of the faithful in an incorruptible body (1 Cor 15:52-54; Acts 23:6; 24:15), eternal life (Tit 1:2; 3:7), seeing God and being conformed to his likeness (1 Jn 3:2f). New Testament hope therefore is said to stabilize the soul like an anchor by linking it to God's steadfastness (Heb 3:6; 6:18-19), and produces the moral fruits of joyful confidence in God (Rom 8:28), unashamed patience in tribulation (Rom 5:3) and perseverance in prayer.

The Basis of New Testament Hope Is the Resurrection of Jesus Christ
As Peter says in his first epistle, "God has given us new birth into a living hope through the resurrection of Jesus Christ from the dead" (1 Pet 1:3). So the basis of the New Testament hope is God's past activity in Jesus Christ who reveals God's purpose for his whole creation. We hope in confidence because Jesus has inaugurated the kingdom and has been raised from the dead. On this basis, the believer looks forward to the resurrection of God's people and the arrival of God's kingdom. We can pray "Thy kingdom come" and celebrate the Lord's Supper in anticipation of the heavenly banquet because we look back to Christ's death and resurrection which open

the way to the kingdom (1 Cor 11:26). In a community with others, we experience the Spirit as a foretaste of the eschatological kingdom (2 Cor 1:22). Through the Spirit, we also receive a super abundance of hope (Rom 15:13). For this reason, Paul calls Jesus Christ "our hope" (1 Tim 1:1; cf. Col 1:27). Because he has risen as the "first fruits," we shall also all rise (1 Cor 15:20-22). The resurrection of Jesus is the basis of our hope that an "Easter" lies ahead at the end of our own history.

The New Testament hope is also based on the promise of the return of Jesus Christ. *Parousia* as the basis of our hope is in the minds of both Peter and Paul. "Set your hope fully on the grace to be given you when Jesus Christ is revealed" (1 Pet 1:13). Paul in a similar tone, says, "The grace of God that brings salvation has appeared . . . . It teaches us . . . to live . . . in this present age, while we wait for the blessed hope—the glorious appearing of our great God and Saviour, Jesus Christ" (Tit 2:11-13).

The Nature of New Testament Hope Is a Living Hope
Because the New Testament Christian hope is based on the resurrected Christ, the apostle Peter calls this hope "a living hope." Peter makes it clear that the nature of New Testament hope is a living one, because it arises from a living relationship with Jesus Christ. When a commitment is made to Jesus Christ, the Spirit of Christ, the Holy Spirit makes the New Testament hope real in our lives. In Romans 15:13, Paul prays, "May the God of hope fill you with all joy and peace as you trust in him, so that you may overflow with hope by the power of the Holy Spirit."

The Purpose of New Testament Hope Is to Shape the Christian Character
In his first epistle to the Thessalonian church, Paul says: "We continually remember before our God the Father your work produced by faith, your labour prompted by love, and your endurance inspired by hope in our Lord Jesus Christ" (1 Thess 1:3). This suggests that the purpose of Christian hope is to shape the Christian character for every aspect of the Christian life. Clearly, this verse suggests an intimate and reciprocal relationship among the three theological virtues: faith, love, and hope. But in other parts of Paul's writing, he sees the Christian hope contribute both to the fruit of the Spirit as

summarized in Galatians 5:22-23 and other desirable attributes of Christian life. As Paul explains, hope brings joy (Rom 5:2), confidence (Rom 5:4), boldness (2 Cor 3:12), freedom (Rom 8:21), and peace (Rom 5:1-3). Hope also motivates Christians for personal purity (1 Jn 3:3) and spurs us on to strive for holiness (Heb 12:14). It gives strength and courage since it protects the inner man as a helmet protects the head (1 Thess 5:8).

In Paul's teaching, it is not only that hope builds Christian character, the converse is also true in that the development of character leads to the strengthening of our hope. In Romans, Paul states that "we rejoice in the hope of the glory of God. Not only so, but we also rejoice in our sufferings, because we know that suffering produces perseverance; perseverance, character; and character, hope" (Rom 5:2-4). Paul sees the positive side of suffering in that he sees that the end result for us is that our hope in God will be greater than before the suffering. It is surely for this reason that Paul encourages believers to "give thanks in all circumstances, for this is God's will for you in Christ Jesus" (1 Thess 5:18) or "Rejoice in the Lord always. I will say it again: Rejoice!" (Phil 4:4). The rationale for this is not any form of masochism, but is the sort of character formation that suffering brings, trusting in the hope of God. And this should lead to a welling up of joy and hope in God's mercy and grace.

Hope in the Traditions of the Church

It would be fair to characterize the hope of the early church fathers as primarily revolutionary and other-worldly and often expressed in apocalyptic terms with judgment, followed by a new and final order of all creation. Augustine may be held responsible for the perpetuation of this conventional form of hope. In City of God and elsewhere, he expresses great pessimism about human history and civilization. He also depicts the city of God and the earthly city as social and political entities which are locked in conflict within the world and within history. Quite naturally he sees Christian life as countercultural and hope is essentially focused on a transcendent heavenly future (i.e., otherworldly). And this form of Christian hope was to be entertained by most Christians down to the present time.

Eighteenth-century Enlightenment however, has brought with it a new interpretation of eschatology. Instead of the more apocalyptic and revolutionary interpretations, Enlightenment thinkers adopted the more evolutionary view of eschatology. Immanuel Kant's view is representative of thinkers of the Enlightenment period. In his view, religion has moved through three stages: the Jewish faith, which was replaced by the Christian faith in its ecclesiastical form, which is to be gradually replaced by a purely rational/moral religion. To Kant this is God's kingdom, and when it finally establishes itself, "the very form of a church is dissolved, the viceroy [Christ] becomes at one with man who is raised up to his level as a citizen of heaven, and so God is all in all."[14]

Immanuel Kant was influential in shaping liberal theology of the nineteenth century both in Europe and in America. For example, in Albrecht Ritschl's theology, the Kingdom of God is understood as a this-worldly moral ideal to be gradually realized with the state as a means to the kingdom. This liberal eschatology, in attempting to accommodate to the cultural and intellectual climate of the time, departed so far from biblical eschatology that it virtually eliminated the apocalyptic notes of judgment and renewal.

It is so totally foreign to Jesus' understanding of the kingdom that one twentieth-century theologian remarked that "the real difference between our modern Protestant worldview and that of primitive Christianity is that we do not share the eschatological attitude. We pass our lives in the joyful confidence that this world will more and more become the showplace of the people of God."[15] This ethical gradualist version of eschatology became a strand in the social gospel which evoked the famous but scathing remark comment from Richard Niebuhr: "A God without wrath brought men without sin into a kingdom without judgment through the ministrations of a Christ without a cross."[16] It is now a question whether Christianity can recapture the real biblical eschatology which had disappeared in the eighteenth and nineteenth centuries. But to review the twentieth-century eschatologies as expounded by Barth, Pannenberg, and Moltmann will be beyond the scope of this paper. What we are interested to do here is to see how this Enlightenment eschatology has influenced the development of modern medicine.

Medical Technology as a Modern Human's Hope

The basic framework for modern medicine was established around the nineteenth century on the foundation of the modern sciences of physics, biochemistry, and biology. This biomedical approach to medicine has led to a radically new conceptualization of the human body which is essentially reduced to biochemical and biophysical processes. In the course of this development, the machine becomes the leading metaphor for the human body[17] and technology becomes the backbone of medicine. This understanding of the human being and medicine has undoubtedly provided a great impetus for the great technical progress in medicine. But a great price has to be paid because as a result, medicine is under the grips of medical technology so much so that one writer remarks that "technology is constituent to the type of medicine which prevails today."[18]

Concomitant with this mechanicalization of human body and technologization of medicine, there is what one theologian remarks as "a dilution of the religious valency of the reality of this world . . . ."[19] With this dilution of the religious dimension of reality and secularization of the world, the transcendent dimension of reality and the eschatological hope beyond earthly existence becomes at best an academic hypothesis, while the "here and now" becomes real. As one commentator notes, "In our culture the body is made sacred and salvation of the body comes instead of salvation of the soul."[20] In the modern world, health and medicine are not only of supreme value, they become the sole content of humanity's hope. They have become the most popular religion of this era. In this view, the Kingdom of God is a perfect society made possible by science and technology and individual eternal life is realized by complete health made possible by medicine. Furthermore, with the secularization of medicine and absolutization of human health, modern people develop a distorted (mythologized) expectation from medical technology. This is because living in a materialistic, "here and now" worldview, there is a tendency that "the limitations and vulnerability of human existence as being a bodily existence are not fully accepted"[21] and people attempt to exercise full control over life and health and even wish to exclude death from life through the instrumentality of medical technology. This mythologization of technology accounts for modern people's total obsession with medical progress and development. Understanding the development of modern technology as a part of the secularizing process of modernity alerts us to the need, as Christians in medical professions, to critically evaluate the technological bias of our time. To this end, we now turn to the relationship between technology and value.

Technology and Value

Most philosophers and scientists want to believe that technology in itself is value-neutral and morality comes into play only in its employment. This sort of optimism is apparently also shared by Christian thinkers, as seen in J. Feinberg and P. Feinberg who boldly assert that "misusing technology for evil is not logically inevitable."[22] The assumption here is that technology is neither moral nor immoral, but amoral, and technologies will always remain only as options whose usage is to be decided by human values. But such a view contradicts human experience. One only needs to recall how stethoscope and laparoscope, CAT scans and MRIs, prenatal screening and genetic counselling, etc., have all been introduced initially as options, but subsequently have become socially enforced procedures. In other words, new technologies do not always remain as options; instead they determine our options by shaping our values. As Neil Postman points out in his insightful analysis, technologies change subtly the society's definition of "knowing" and "truth," and "alter those deeply embedded habits of thought which give to a culture its sense of what the world is like—a sense of what is the natural order of things, of what is reasonable, of what is necessary, of what is inevitable, of what is real."[23] This is so because intrinsic in every technology is an ideological bias which subtly predisposes one to see the world in one way and not the other, and to value one thing over another. It should be borne in mind that medical technologies do not only service medicine, they also shape our medical ideologies, values, and practices.

With the advent of genetic technology, one has good reason to be concerned that this technology will ultimately redefine what human nature is. From the perspective of genetic technology, human beings have become DNA and control over the DNA therefore provides the opportunity to exercise control over the human being and her destiny. But we must not think of this as a kind of conspiracy planned by the technocrats, with the patients as totally unwilling victims; rather, modern patients as medical consumers have contributed a great deal in reinforcing this form of technological imperative by supporting and demanding that technology. Modern consumers have subscribed to the Enlightenment philosophical premise construction that knowledge is power over nature, and power over nature means human welfare. Following Francis Bacon, most modern people accept the axiom that science and technology are necessary sources of progress which we must have, and choose to ignore the controlling power such technology may exercise over our lives. This is the climax of the sad vision that C. S. Lewis wrote about in *The Abolition of Man* when he said that "what we call man's power over Nature [technology] turns out to be a power exercised by some men over other men with Nature [technology] as its instrument."[24]

Technology, then, far from being value-neutral, is value-laden, and is possessive of a power which shapes human values and controls medical practices. It both legitimates and authorizes people to do certain things and not others, a role which, not too long ago, was usually reserved for God. In the pre-modern days, when people of the West still retained their belief in God, the society lived by the principle that all the goodness that knowledge and technology brought ultimately came from God and so all knowledge and technology must reflect God's goodness and must be directed to glorify God. Such a theology provides order and meaning to human existence, stipulates the limits and purpose for technology and progress, and protects the society from the tyranny and the subordinating power of technology. Much of modern society's abuse of and confusion about medicine stems from the fact that it has allowed theology to be replaced by technology as its controlling ideology. Christians must therefore rectify this situation by bringing medical technology once again under the guidance of a biblical theology of creation, providence, stewardship, and eschatology, wherein our Christian hope lies.

Creation and Providence

Larry Rasmussen has rightly reminded us that "creation" is a theological term and not a biblical term, and the verb form "creating" is more consistently used in the Bible.[25] This open nature of "creating" implies God's continuing activity in sustaining the world which he has brought into being (Ps 104:27; Gen 8:22). It means that were God to withdraw his sustaining providence, the world would perish. This is consistent with the biblical meaning of divine providence which, understood correctly, means that the Creator sustains and rules over what he has already brought into being in the initial creation (Mt 10:29; Ps 113: 5, 6). While this view of divine providence underlines the radical contingency of the world upon God, it does not mean that the creation is thereby closed to all new possibilities and the future is wholly determined by the present; what it does emphasize is that whatever new possibilities we may anticipate, they are entirely dependent on the mercy of God, so that creation's openness is ultimately an openness to the goodness and sovereignty of God. Regrettably, some theologians have misunderstood creation's openness to mean the unfinished character of the cosmos and human beings as co-creators to finish God's unfinished business. Cole-Turner for example sees the Human Genome Project as an opportunity to expand our ability to participate in God's work of continuing creation.[26] But there is no biblical basis for understanding God's creation as unfinished. The Bible speaks of the stability and actuality of the original creation, which is evidenced by the institution of the Sabbath (Gen 1, 2; Ps 93:1, 102:25; Is 45:11-12). And correspondingly, it is incorrect to think of God's providence as a kind of continuous creation (*creatio continua*) and human's participation in it as co-creators. Rather a biblical understanding of the openness of creation denies the self-containing and self-sufficient nature of the created world and reminds us of the continuing providential care of the Holy Spirit who from the beginning has been present (Gen 1:2).[27] An open system of creation therefore emphasizes the total dependence upon God and his goodness, and creation can be called "good" only to the extent that through it the goodness of the Creator is manifested and experienced, and not due to any of its intrinsic goodness, actual or potential. This suggests that whatever else the goodness of creation means, in order for creation to be good, it should exist and function in such a way that it fulfils the Creator's intention and purpose for creation, which is communion, relationship, and love; this intention of communion in turn reflects the goodness of the Creator, the triune God who in eternity is communion, relationship, and love.

Man, Nature, and Stewardship

Fundamental behind modern society's development of technology is its distorted perception of the goodness of the creation and hence its uneasy relationship with creation. To most modern people, creation or nature is the enemy and a threat to human welfare; science and technology is the only way to enable humanity to progress and to triumph over nature. But as embodied beings created out of dust, human beings are too much part of nature to allow such a presumptuous triumphalistic posture. We may transcend nature in certain important ways, but our embodied state is connected to and dependent on nature, and may never live simply "over against" nature. A more biblical approach puts human beings not over, nor under, but within nature. But to embrace nature and to reject modern society's triumphalistic perspective is not to adopt an anti-technological spirit. Embodied persons are children of nature as much as children of spirit, and as the image of God, the Creator's stewards, we have been given the mandate to exercise dominion on nature: to fill, to rule, and to care for the land. While this does not preclude the development and employment of technology, it does imply that both its development and employment ought to be brought under the guidance of biblical stewardship.

We should now reflect on these three aspects of human stewardship in the context of the development and employment of medical technology. Reichenbach and Anderson interpret the mandate to fill the land in a qualitative sense, and sees the injunction as a warrant, in the name of human betterment, to engage in genetic engineering, including germ-line cell manipulation, in order to re-design human beings that are genetically and intellectually more superior.[28] But are stewards called to improve upon creation? And if so, how? To improve by repairing certain genetic defects is obviously different from redesigning certain genetic structures. Some would believe that the mandate to rule, a word which in its original Hebrew form does connote the sense of absolute subjugation, empowers human stewards to do whatever they can through technology. But as Reichenbach and Anderson themselves have pointed out, the mandate to rule should be qualified by two considerations:

1. The power to rule is not self-derived, but delegated
2. The power to rule the creation should therefore be consistent

with the intention and purpose of the Creator for the creation[29]

This, together with the explicit mandate "to take care of the land"
(Gen 2:15) which is understood to mean serving, preserving, guard-
ing, protecting, cultivating, and benefiting, could only lead to the
conclusion that we are called to be accountable stewards.

Modern society places the stewardly functions given to humans
in a context different from the biblical times. Whereas in the pre-
modern era, the natural environment was a constant threat to human existence and survival, now the table has been turned around,
with the environment being exploited and devastated. Similarly, not
too long ago, humans fell victims to the fragility of their bodily functions, now they are equipped with such technology that they can
control the body and even re-design its composition. In this context,
technology has the potential to elevate human beings from stewards
to gods, i.e., to perform tasks that properly only belong to God and
to change what only God has the right to change. But God's stewards should not play God, but be accountable to God.

To be accountable stewards, Reichenbach and Anderson suggest
that we need to consider five important and difficult questions and
we may apply these considerations in our reflections on medical
technology in general, and genetic technology in particular:

1. What are we obligated to change?
2. Are changes permissible or obligatory?
3. For what purpose are we to change creation?
4. What are the limits of the change?
5. What are the limits of the risks of any proposed change?[30]

Even if we accept the premise that to be God's steward involves a
moral injunction to change certain parts of the creation which may
include battling diseases, controlling floods, reducing pollutions,
etc., we still wonder whether the obligation to change includes direct
alteration of human nature such as the genetic composition in order
to produce a new human being who is genetically and intellectually
more superior and more able to adapt to the environment. It is very
questionable whether this kind of improvement can be justified in
view of the alteration of human genetic composition it entails. Stewardship should be guided by a purpose which is clearly in line with
the purpose and intention of the Creator for the creation. In other

words, our criteria for the legitimacy of any proposed change should be that it facilitates the fulfilment of God's purpose(s) of the creation. As we have alluded to earlier, Reform theology affirms that God creates out of love in order that creation may enjoy the fellowship with God whose triune life is one of communion, relationship, and love. If relationship and communion is the essential nature of God, and consequently the nature of created image of God, then the function of the image, i.e., stewardship must be exercised for the improvement of relationships. On this view, we are obligated to change and improve upon any part of the creation which clearly frustrates the intention of the Creator for relationships with God, fellow stewards and the rest of the creation, and we are limited to undertake any changes which may undermine or have the potential risk to undermine our dependence on God and our interdependence on fellow human beings and the rest of the creation. This means that as God's stewards, not everything that can be done should be done. God sets limits as well as limits to risks. From the tree in the Garden of Eden before the Fall to human mortality after the Fall, God has always imposed limits on his own creatures, including human beings and their achievement (Gen 11). This strongly suggests that there are certain things only God can do and achieve, and these should not be attempted even by human's almighty technology.

Conclusion

To conclude, we are reminded of Thomas Aquinas' teaching of the two sins against hope: despair and presumption. In the *Summa Theologica*, Aquinas taught that there are two kinds of despair. The first kind arises because of "a distaste for spiritual things, and not to hope for them as arduous goods."[31] Western modern society clearly committed this error when it decided to remove all theological underpinnings from its post-Christian secular anthropology. Aquinas further suggested that the second source of despair arises from a lack of confidence in the infinite goodness of God. When the modern West chose to place its hope in science and technology, it allowed the goodness of God's intention for communion, fellowship, relationship, and love to be replaced by conquest, control, manipulation, and exploitation. When genuine hope in God, guaranteed by the resurrection of the Son Jesus Christ, is lost in the horizon of human vision of progress, modern people have lost what the author of Hebrews called the "anchor for the soul" and fallen in a state of despair unprecedented in human history. How else can one explain a society's maddening quest for technological advances to cure diseases and to extend life, and at the same time advocates with an equally frantic passion to end lives with euthanasia and assisted suicide?

The second sin people may commit against hope, according to Aquinas, is presumption, which in contrast to despair, which presupposes non-fulfilment of God's promises, assumes the condition of fulfilment. Modern people commit the sin of presumption by relying on their own power to achieve the promises of God. We sin against the divine character of hope by assuming that we are able to create a "new heaven and new earth" and to fulfil God's promises of eternal blessing by human achievement through the power of technology. As Aquinas comments, "Such like presumption seems to arise directly from pride, for it is owing to a great desire for glory, that a man attempts things beyond his power . . . ."[32] Modern medicine needs to repent of its sin of despair and presumption, and relocate itself in the Christian resurrection hope which is the "anchor for the soul, firm and secure" (Heb 6:19).

Notes

[1] J. Robert Nelson, ed., *Life as Liberty, Life as Trust* (Grand Rapids, Mich.: Eerdmans, 1992), 84.

[2] Vaclav Havel, *Disturbing the Peace* (New York: Vintage, 1991), 181.

[3] Desmond Tutu, *Hope and Suffering* (Grand Rapids, Mich.: Eerdmans, 1984).

[4] For an excellent discussion of the relationship between trust and hope, see Arthur A. Vogel's *God's Presence in Man's World* (London: Geoffrey Chapman, 1973), ch. 4.

[5] A. T. Beck, *Depression: Cause and Treatment* (Philadelphia: University of Pennsylvania Press, 1967), 58, in *Baker's Encyclopedia of Psychology*, ed. David G. Benner (Grand Rapids, Mich.: Baker Book House, 1985), 528.

[6] David Aikman, *Hope: The Heart's Great Quest* (Ann Arbor, Mich.: Vine Books, 1995), 12–13.

[7] Michael F. Scheier and C. S. Carver, "Dispositional Optimism and Recovery from Coronary Bypass Surgery: The Beneficial Effects on Physical and Psychological Well-being," *Journal of Personality and Social Psychology*, 57 (1987): 1024–

40; quoted by Aikman, *Hope*, 13.

[8] E. Bloch, "Prinzip der Hoffnung" (Frankfurt, Germany: Suhrkamp, 1959), 284-85, quoted in John Macquarrie, *In Search of Humanity* (New York: Crossroad, 1989), 244.

[9] E. Bloch, *Man on His Own* (New York: E. T. Herder & Herder, 1970), 152.

[10] Havel, *Disturbing the Peace*, 181.

[11] For the following discussion on the Jewish tradition, I am indebted to the excellent summary provided by Aikman in his *Hope: The Heart's Great Quest.*

[12] All scriptural quotations in this article are taken from the New International version of the Bible, copyright the New York International Bible Society.

[13] Milton Steinberg, *Basic Judaism* (New York: Harcourt, Brace & Co. 1965), 53.

[14] Immanuel Kant, *Religion within the Limits of Reason Alone*, trans. T. M. Green and H. H. Hudson (New York: Harper & Row, 1960), 126.

[15] Johannes Weiss, *Jesus' Proclamation of the Kingdom of God*, trans. R. H. Hiers and D. L. Holland (London: S. C. M. Press, 1971), 135.

[16] Richard Niebuhr, *The Kingdom of God in America* (New York: Harper Torchbooks, 1959), 193.

[17] H. Jochemsen et al., "The Medical Profession in Modern Society: The Importance of Defining Limits" in *Bioethics and the Future of Medicine: A Christian Appraisal*, ed. John F. Kilner, Nigel M. de S. Cameron, and David L. Schiedermayer (Grand Rapids, Mich.: Eerdmans, 1995), 15.

[18] Have H. Ten and G. Wackers, "In de greep van de medische technologie (In the grip of medical technology)," *Wijsgerig Perspektiefi* 28 , no. 3(1987/8): 890-95; quoted in H. Jochemsen et al., "The Medical Profession in Modern Society," 25 n.11.

[19] Romano Guardini, *Religie en openbaring (Religion and Revelation)* (Hilversum, Netherlands: P. Brand, 1963), 32; quoted in ibid., 25 n.16.

[20] J. Rolies, "Gezondheid: een nieuwe religie? (Health: A New Religion?)," in *De gezonde burger (The Healthy Citizen)*, ed. J. Rolies (Nijmegen, Netherlands: Sun, 1988), 24; quoted in ibid., 26 n.18.

[21] H. Jochemsen et al., "The Medical Profession in Modern Society," 16.

[22] J. Feinberg and P. Feinberg, *Ethics for a Brave New World* (Wheaton, Ill.: Crossway Books, 1993), 290.

[23] Neil Postman, *Technopoly: The Surrender of Culture to Technology* (New York: Vintage Books, 1993), 12.

[24] C. S. Lewis, *The Abolition of Man* (London: HarperCollins Publishing, 1978), 35.

[25] Larry Rasmussen, "Creation, Church, and Christian Responsibility," in *Tending the Garden*, ed. Wesley Granberg-Michaelson (Grand Rapids, Mich.: Eerdmans, 1987), 116.

[26] R. Cole-Turner, *The New Genesis: Theology and the Genetic Revolution* (Westminster, England: John Knox Press, 1993).

27 James M. Houston, *I Believe in the Creator* (Grand Rapids, Mich.: Eerdmans, 1980), 105.

28 Bruce R. Reichenbach and V. Elving Anderson, *On Behalf of God: A Christian Ethic for Biology* (Grand Rapids, Mich.: Eerdmans, 1995), 50–51.

29 Ibid., 52.

30 Ibid., 56–66.

31 Thomas Aquinas, *Summa Theologia*, II-II, Q.20 art. 4, trans. Fathers of the English Dominican Province (Westminster, England: Christian Classic, 1981), 1256.

32 Ibid., II-II, Q. 21, art. 4, 1258.

Robert O. Stephens

When Is Enough, Enough?

Several months ago I shared a delicious breakfast at a downtown Vancouver hotel with Dr. Hui and a few others in order to lay plans for this conference. Dr. Hui suggested, and we all agreed, that as part of the Conference we would need to discuss issues related to death and dying. The conversation then turned to whom might handle such a topic and all eyes turned in my direction. I felt honoured but a bit apprehensive as I considered this request.

I am sure that the reasoning behind this unanimity lay not in my scholarship or erudition, but in the fact that I was by far the oldest in the group, had white hair and very probably would be the first one in the group to face the reality of death. I suppose too that having enjoyed the practice of medicine for nearly fifty years I had seen more people die than anyone in the group, especially during the decade I spent in Central Africa as a medical missionary.

It was when I was in my early teens that I first gave any thought to the meaning of death; not that I was morbid or gave it a great deal of consideration. Like most teenagers I was more interested in getting on with life, than thinking about death. However I was studying piano at the time and my teacher gave me a chorale by Bach to learn to play entitled *Komm Süsser Tod*—"Come, Sweet Death." It was a lovely, quiet, sombre melody with a very soft ending. As a teenager I puzzled over the title—how could death be sweet? It seemed to me then that death would more likely be bitter than sweet. It has taken me a lifetime to work through the answer, and I am still learning.

Perhaps another reason that the breakfast group asked me to deal with this topic is that an older person has experienced firsthand some of the realities of the normal ageing process which leads to progressive impairment of function and inevitably to death. Jean

Paul Sartre the existential philosopher wrote that "The meaning of life is found in death." More recently the well-known psychiatrist Ernest Becker in his book entitled *The Denial of Death* wrote in the preface:

> The prospect of death wonderfully concentrates the mind. The main thesis of this book is that it does much more than that: the idea of death, the fear of it, haunts the human animal like nothing else; it is the main-spring of human activity—activity designed largely to avoid the fatality of death, to overcome it by denying in some way that it is the final destiny for man.[1]

The ever-increasing popularity of Grecian hair formula, cremes to remove wrinkles, and plastic surgeons to eliminate crow's feet and double chins indicate man's, and woman's, continuing desire to suppress the reality of death. The quest for the fountain of youth and immortality continues unabated.

In contrast, the Scriptures remind us clearly of the reality and inevitability of death. "For as in Adam all die," says St. Paul (1 Cor 15:22).[2] "Man is destined to die once" says the writer to the Hebrews (Heb 9:27).

I can attest to the reality of the normal ageing process. Every summer I play a few games of golf. Despite switching to steel "woods" and extra-lively balls, my drives now fall far short of where they used to drop. If I play eighteen holes, I use an electric cart otherwise gross muscle fatigue overtakes me. And if I play on a hilly course I am slower climbing the hills, more breathless when I reach the summits, and my cardiac rate is noticeably higher. When I get in the rough and scratch my leg, the healing process takes considerably longer than before. All these changes indicate a normal physiological decline in my bodily functions.

I know too from studies that have been reported using CAT scanning and MRI that my brain size is decreasing, my cerebral ventricles and sulci are enlarging, and that the number of my neuronal synaptic connections are steadily decreasing.

Despite all these changes, I would make a plea to the younger generations that they do not write off those of us who are over seventy. In this connection I note that Bill Bright, the dynamic founder of Campus Crusade for Christ, has recently received the prestigious

Templeton Prize for Progress in Religion. He is now seventy-four.

Certainly, as health care providers we should do all we can to as-sist our patients through the inevitable changes of ageing. Advice regarding lifestyle changes related to diet, weight, smoking, stress, cholesterol, exercise, etc., should be carefully given. However when one examines survival curves, while more people are living longer than they were in the early part of this century, with rare exceptions, no one is living beyond one hundred years of age, which was also the case a century ago. In other words, we have increased the percentage of people approaching the biological limit, but we have not in-creased the limit.

At the point when age and physical and mental disabilities reach a certain threshold we must consider whether certain interventions should be attempted. A threshold of about age sixty is accepted for cardiac or bone marrow transplants. A threshold somewhere in the eighties is appropriate for aortic valve replacement. It is important for us to assess and accept the limitations of disease and the ageing process—to know when enough is enough.

The patient, the family, and the health care team must all be in-volved in making such decisions. When it is decided that the patient will live out the natural history of the disease, then all those involved must affirm this decision, accept the inevitable, and strive to make the remaining time as pleasant as possible. Second-guessing whatever decision has been made should be avoided but rather a warm, lov-ing, and supportive environment should be provided. In this con-nection Mother Theresa has stated:

> The biggest disease today is not Leprosy or Tuberculo-sis, but rather the feeling of being unwanted, uncared for, and deserted by everybody. The greatest evil is lack of love, the terrible indifference—towards one's neigh-bours who live at the roadside assaulted by exploitation, poverty, and diseases.
>
> The unwanted are hungry not for food but for love; they are thirsty not for water but for peace; they are na-ked not for clothes but for dignity; they are homeless not for shelter but for understanding.
>
> You may think your efforts do not count. We our-selves feel that what we are doing is just a drop in the

ocean. But if that drop was not in the ocean I think the ocean will be less because of that missing drop. Even your feeble efforts will bear much fruit if you bring God into your life. If you can love and share, you will be happy, genuinely so.

Finally, in this connection, I would like to quote from a recent editorial in the Journal of the Society of Obstetricians and Gynaecologists of Canada by Dr. Stephen Genuis, a participant at this Conference. Dr. Genuis is a CMDS member who has written widely. He is Associate Clinical Professor at the University of Alberta in Edmonton.

> The end stages of a person's life have the potential to be immensely important. It is a time when forgiveness can be offered and received, hurt relationships can be restored, when the opportunity for tenderness and sharing is often facilitated, and when love and leave-taking may be communicated in a unique way. Over the last number of years, increasing numbers of individuals and groups have spoken of and lobbied for the concept of "death with dignity." However, one must question if as individuals, professional groups, and society we are in danger of shifting our priorities away from the more important issue. With increasing attention being directed towards various forms of euthanasia, we risk losing sight of the need to provide better and more effective care for individuals and their families at the end of life. The real issue worthy of emphasis is not "death with dignity" but rather the need to facilitate "life with dignity."[3]

Of course we are all too well aware that one alternative being suggested to such life with dignity is physician-assisted death or assisted suicide or mercy killing.

The debate in Canada regarding this alternative may very well heat up in the months to come especially in light of two recent court decisions in the United States which have thrown the door wide open to physician-assisted suicide. On March 6, 1996, the Ninth Circuit Federal Court of Appeals said terminally ill patients have a constitutional right to physician-assisted suicide. Two days later, a jury in Michigan acquitted Dr. Jack Kevorkian of assisting suicide. The first ruling will now allow states to legalize physician-assisted suicide.[4] The second ruling further weakens the moral barriers to suicide and will fuel the pro-death movement.

The ruling by the Ninth Circuit Court was brazen in that it founded its arguments on the discovery of a "a constitutionally-protected liberty interest in determining the time and manner of one's own death."[5] The autonomy argument which has been used to defend the right to abortion and which pro-life forces have tried to use to defend the unborn is here used to defend the right to assisted suicide. The United States may well follow the course of Holland which has allowed physician-assisted suicide for over a decade. A recent Dutch government study discovered that over half the patients killed never requested death. Can we be far behind?

Should anyone be in doubt about the nature of our ruling elite the US decision should dispel those uncertainties. Prof. Alasdair MacIntyre said in 1991 that

> they [the barbarians] are not waiting beyond our frontiers; they have already been governing us for quite sometime. And it is our lack of consciousness of this that constitutes part of our predicament.[6]

A Canadian professor of Law, M. H. Ogilvie, has described our rulers as "elites plundering their spiritual inheritance." Camus spoke of "the death instinct at work in our society."

The hard questions must now be answered. Can medicine embrace these ideas and be unchanged in the process? I believe the answer is now clearly no. Does the "death instinct" dominate the profession? I think the answer is again no but a significant proportion will embrace it. Is the Hippocratic, Judeo-Christian tradition important to preserve? I think the answer is yes for anyone who accepts the traditional Christian view of human nature. One has only to see the fearful relationship that exists between patient and healer in pagan societies where the healer may also kill, to understand how precious was the gift that Hippocrates gave and the church built into our culture.

The Christian Medical and Dental Society of Canada has taken a clear stand against physician participation, whether direct or indirect, in assisted suicide. Principles and observations regarding euthanasia from a Christian perspective have been clearly stated in our paper submitted to the Special Senate Committee on Euthanasia and Assisted Suicide. Hopefully this submission had some impact on the Committee's decision not to recommend legislation supporting euthanasia. The battle may have been won but I suspect the war will continue. Traditionally a physician has provided care for two reasons: to sustain life and to relieve suffering. In assisted suicide the primary purpose of the treatment is to cause death. Such a purpose has no role in the professional responsibilities of a physician. From the time of Hippocrates physicians have been instructed to refuse their patients' request for death-causing treatments.

I am concerned, too, regarding the impact on the medical profession if doctors were trained and authorized to kill, even for reasons of the utmost mercy and compassion. When US physicians offered to carry out capital punishment by lethal injection there was a great public outcry expressing abhorrence at physicians being agents of death, even if it were legal.

In the face of increasing pressure to legalize physician assisted suicide what can we do? Our sister Society, CMDS-US suggests the following:

> *Pray* that God will turn the hearts of the people of our nation to Jesus Christ and His principles to guide us through life and death.
>
> *Speak out* on this vital issue by letting your legislators know your views.
>
> *Reach out* with true compassion to the elderly, handicapped, and seriously ill. Let them know that you care and that a loving God has a purpose for their lives.[7]

Secondly, I believe we should put increasing emphasis on the hospice alternative and particularly on the Christian hospice alternative. We should bend every effort to find increasingly effective methods of relieving physical pain, nausea, constipation, and insomnia. We must provide effective support for mental, psychological, financial, and spiritual distress.

In fact, as the pressure for physician assisted suicide increases, it may well require us to begin again the cycle of establishing Christian hospitals—centres of healing which address the needs of the whole person based on Christian principles and from a Christian perspective. In this connection, an interesting and innovative model is being developed in Winnipeg. It is outlined and discussed in the May 1996 issue of *Focus*, the quarterly magazine of CMDS Canada.

At this point it is appropriate to consider the distinction between physician-assisted suicide and foregoing life-sustaining treatment. In the former the intention is death, in the latter the intention is to stop postponing inevitable death. Enough is enough. In the former there is an attitude of arrogance, in the latter one of humility. In the former the means of death is killing and the agent the physician. In the latter the means of death is withholding or withdrawing treatment and the agent is the disease itself.

There are at least three positions that one can espouse in regard to these issues. On the one extreme are those who espouse the radical right to self-determination because in their view individual freedom is the highest good. This is the "right-to-die" or the "right-to-choose" group. They view stopping treatment as passive euthanasia which they accept along with active forms.

On the other extreme are those who espouse the radical "right-to-life" position which views cessation of treatment as euthanasia which to them is quite wrong. They view biological life as the highest good and therefore all treatment must be maintained as long as possible.

Personally, I would maintain a middle ground, that is, compassionate care of the dying which would include the right of the patient to refuse death-postponing treatment. The patient, when ready, may say "enough is enough."

Peter was a long-time friend, neighbour, and patient. He possessed a healthy body, a sharp mind, and a quiet but profound faith in God. His passion was sailing, and he would often invite my wife and I for an afternoon on his boat which was anchored in the Toronto harbour. Summer sailing on Lake Ontario can be an exciting and invigorating experience. A few years before his retirement from a senior business position he began to notice some fatigue. This increased gradually year by year. He had no specific complaints and a thorough physical examination was unremarkable.

He retired, sold his sail boat and stopped playing tennis. He gave up gardening and in fact all activities except those of daily living. He then went into hospital for a minor procedure requiring a light anaesthetic. However the anaesthetist encountered severe difficulties after surgery in getting the patient to breathe on his own. This led to a harder look at the whole situation and eventually a diagnosis of Amyotrophic Lateral Sclerosis (ALS) was established. The patient was allowed to go home but continued to lose strength although his mental faculties remained as sharp as ever.

Eventually he was admitted to hospital, and his continual down-hill course required a tracheotomy for assisted breathing, a gastrotomy for feeding due to his inability to swallow without aspiration, and finally full time on a respirator. He was in hospital for four months.

Peter had always enjoyed good communication with his wife. His time in hospital was no exception. Although Peter could not talk, he communicated clearly through nodding, his eye expression, and his faint grimaces or smiles.

After extensive discussion with the health care team, Peter requested and his wife agreed that the respirator be turned off. This was done late one night and early in the morning Peter passed peacefully into the loving arms of his God—truly a bright and happy morning for him!

Now let us consider more specifically the problem of withdrawal of treatment as related to feeding, hydration, and the persistent vegetative state. As you all understand, this is indeed a thorny issue. I will only touch on some of the highlights and hopefully give some guidelines to help us decide when enough is enough in this area.

Firstly what is persistent vegetative state (PVS)? The Multi-Society Task Force on PVS has given the following definition:

1. No evidence of awareness of self or environment and an inability to interact with others
2. No evidence of sustained, reproducible, purposeful, or voluntary behavioural responses to visual, auditory, tactile, or noxious stimuli
3. No evidence of language comprehension or expression
4. Intermittent wakefulness manifested by the presence of sleep-wake cycles
5. Sufficiently preserved hypothalamic and brain-stem autonomic functions to permit survival with medical and nursing care

6. Bowel and bladder incontinence

7. Variably preserved cranial-nerve reflexes (pupillary, oculo-cephalic, corneal, vestibulo-ocular, and gag) and spinal reflexes[8]

Additionally the wakeful unconscious state must have existed for longer than a few weeks. Also, the time from brain injury to the point of diagnosis must be at least one month.

PVS should not be confused with patients dying from terminal cancer or AIDS or who have suffered a recent stroke or cardiac arrest. Further, PVS should not be confused with brain death which is the complete absence of brain function, including the brainstem. A brain dead person requires a ventilator. In a case of brain death, most Christian ethicists believe that families have no moral obligation to maintain their relative on a ventilator or in intensive care. Finally, PVS should not be confused with the "Locked-in Syndrome" in which consciousness and cognition are maintained but movement and communication are impossible because of severe motor paralysis. Although rare, this syndrome is compatible with prolonged survival.

Statistically, over 90% of patients with coma either from traumatic or non-traumatic head injury will recover or die within one month. Also the majority of patients in PVS recover or die by one year after the injury. Even among those who survive for one year the mortality is high. Chances of survival beyond fifteen years are remote—perhaps 1:50,000.

A very difficult area of discussion for Christians is the issue of withdrawal of food and water from a patient with PVS. Unfortunately no Scripture speaks directly to this issue.

Religious opinion regarding discontinuing medical care varies in our culture. Orthodox Jewish opinion is most firmly against any discontinuation of supportive care. In a paper published in 1990 a panel of Catholic theologians made the following statement:

> We see withholding nutrition or hydration as passive euthanasia and morally offensive if the intention was to directly kill the patient by this means. However, if the intention was to remove the patient from unusual, gravely burdensome, extraordinary or futile medical intervention, with the foreseen but unintended conse-

quence that death would come more quickly, this
would be understood as a legitimate allowing-to-die and
would not be considered euthanasia, either active or
passive.[9]

Clearly the Catholic view makes the motive of those making the decision the key element in the determination of moral culpability.

Mainline Protestant views have centred on patient autonomy,
and the futility of certain therapies. In an article in the *Journal of
Neurological Sciences*, E. V. Spudis states "No Christian is obliged to
prolong life indefinitely, nor should he even try. Medicalizing technology to prolong life indefinitely is as futile as it is obscene."[10]

Finally, our sister society in the United States has published a
position paper on tube feeding which I would now like to quote to
you. Although we have no similar paper in Canada, I suspect that
our position would mirror that of our US counterparts' "The Withholding or Withdrawing of Nutrition and Hydration":

> The primary goal of the Christian clinical ethic is to
> provide compassionate medical care to all human be-
> ings. We recognize that nutritional support is both a
> universal human biologic requirement and a funda-
> mental demonstration of human caring. Because we be-
> lieve that there should be a basic covenant between all
> of us to care for those who are incapacitated, we are
> committed to the provision of food and water to those
> who cannot feed themselves.
>
> In exceptional cases, tube feeding may actually result
> in increased patient suffering during the dying process.
> Although we have a basic covenant to offer food and
> water to patients, we recognize that the provision of en-
> tral or parentral nutrition may not be indicated in pa-
> tients who are clearly and irreversibly deteriorating, who
> are beyond a reasonable hope of recovery, and in whom
> death appears imminent. In such cases, it is ethically
> permissible to withhold or withdraw nutrition and hy-
> dration, in full consideration of patient and family
> wishes.
>
> However, we believe that physicians, other health pro-
> fessionals, and health care facilities should initiate and

continue nutritional support and hydration when their patients cannot feed themselves. We are concerned that demented, severely retarded, and comatose individuals are increasingly viewed as "useless mouths." (We reject the dehumanizing phrase.) Rather than encouraging physicians to withhold or withdraw such patients' food and water, we encourage physicians to respond to God's call for improved physical, social, and spiritual support of all vulnerable human beings.[11]

Personally, I believe that there is a fundamental difference between refusing treatment and being put to death with the assistance of a physician. A patient has the right to refuse treatment and to receive adequate pain relief even if this may shorten life but it is inherently, morally, and legally unacceptable to kill another human being or to assist in intentionally causing death.

In conclusion I would like to consider a passage of Scripture which bears on this subject and introduces additional factors which are very important to consider. It is the story of Jesus and Peter as recorded in the Gospel of Luke 5:1-11.

One day as [Jesus] was standing by the Lake of Gennesaret, with the people crowding around him and listening to the word of God, he saw at the water's edge two boats, left there by the fishermen, who were washing their nets. He got into one of the boats, the one belonging to Simon, and asked him to put out a little from shore. Then he sat down and taught the people from the boat.

When he had finished speaking, he said to Simon, "Put out into deep water, and let down the nets for a catch."

Simon answered, "Master, we've worked hard all night and haven't caught anything. But because you say so, I will let down the nets."

When they had done so, they caught such a large number of fish that their nets began to break. So they signalled their partners in the other boat to come and help them and they came and filled both boats so full that they began to sink.

> When Simon Peter saw this, he fell at Jesus' knees and said, "Go away from me, Lord; I am a sinful man!" For he and all his companions were astonished at the catch of fish they had taken, and so were James and John, the sons of Zebedee, Simon's partners.
>
> Then Jesus said to Simon, "Don't be afraid; from now on you will catch men." So they pulled their boats up on shore, left everything and followed him.

Simon Peter, an expert and experienced professional fisherman had been fishing all night but had caught nothing. He had pulled the boat on shore, and was putting away his nets. He was saying in effect, "enough is enough." He knew all the best spots to fish, all the tricks of the trade, and had worked hard but to no avail. After all, enough is enough. But the Lord asked him to give it one more try. Reluctantly he did so, with miraculous results.

We are expert and experienced dispensers of health care. However sometimes, despite our most valiant efforts, our treatment fails. We are on the point of giving up and packing our medical bag and going home. "Enough is enough." But then the Lord appears and a miracle occurs. He can change the course of events—he can even defy and reverse the statistics or probabilities!

I had an experience of this during my first year as a medical missionary in Zaire, then the Belgian Congo. I began medical work as well as the construction of a hospital in a remote area in Eastern Zaire where no physician had previously worked. The local people were quite wary of this new physician. I prayed that the Lord would intervene to give me and the Gospel credibility.

Obstetrics was a very difficult area of practice. Easy, normal deliveries tended to occur in the villages. Difficult, obstructed cases tended to arrive on my doorstep, often at a very late stage. I knew that I was facing a potentially significantly high rate of maternal mortality. Furthermore, I had no special training in obstetrics. However, in the first year, after more than three hundred deliveries, the maternal mortality rate was zero. My credibility was established but more importantly the credibility of the Gospel. I realized that this was due to the hand of God—a real miracle.

So Peter learned—and I learned—that God can turn a potential failure or disaster into something wonderful. So be careful when you say "enough is enough."

Note also that after the miracle Christ called Peter to give up fishing and follow him. He was to become a fisher of men. After Peter's first sermon recorded in Acts 2, three thousand persons believed. In effect the Lord said to Peter, "Enough is enough—I want you to quit fishing and take up a new phase of life." Peter obeyed, although I believe it was not an easy decision.

I had a similar experience when revolution came to Zaire after I had worked there for more than a decade. Our home, our friends, our work was there. But the Lord said, "Enough is enough." I left Zaire with tears.

But I have long since realized that my experience in Zaire was the basis for an enlarged ministry which the Lord had in store for me. I have learned not to resist or resent when the Lord says "Enough is enough." We should remember this principle as we deal with patients who are facing end of life decisions.

Since leaving Zaire, there have been several occasions in my life when the Lord has rather suddenly changed its course. I know I shall soon have the final one, when he takes me by the hand through the valley of the shadow of death, so that we can enter together the place that he has prepared for me.

I will await with joy that final word, "Come ye blessed of my Father, inherit the Kingdom prepared for you—enough is enough."

Even so come Lord Jesus! And so over the course of a lifetime I have learned the meaning of "Come, sweet death," *Komm Süsser Tod.*

Bibliography

Drain G. et.al. "Assisted Death," *The Lancet* 336 (1990): 610-13.

Fish, A. and Singer P. A. "Nancy B.: The Criminal Code and Decisions to Forgo Life-sustaining Treatment," *Canadian Medical Association Journal* 147, no. 5 (1992): 637-42.

Genuis, S. J., Genuis, S. K., and Chang, W. C. "Public Attitudes Toward the Right to Die," *Canadian Medical Association Journal*, 150, no. 5 (1994): 701-8.

Genuis, S. J., and Genuis, S. K. "Living and Dying with Dignity," *Journal of the Society of Obstetricians and Gynaecologists of Canada* 16, no. 6, (1994): 1771-74.

Genuis, S. J., and Genuis, S. K. "End of Life Decisions; The

Quagmire," *Journal of the Society of Obstetricians and Gynaecologists of Canada* (June 1994): 1809-19.

Genuis, S. J. "Decriminalizing Assisted Suicide; More Than We Bargained For?" *The Medical Post* 30, no. 13 (1994).

Hollman, Jay, ed., *New Issues in Medical Ethics*, Bristol, Tenn.: Christian Medical and Dental Society, 1995.

Hui, Edwin C., ed. *Questions of Right and Wrong*, Vancouver, B.C.: Regent College, 1994.

Orentlicher, David. "Physician Participation in Assisted Suicide," *Journal of the American Medical Association* 262, no. 13 (1989): 1844-45.

Pomerantz, Andrew S. "Death with Dignity: a Right or an Obligation?" *Humane Medicine* 8, no. 1. (1992): 70-73.

Sommerville M. A. "The Harm in Accepting Doctors as Angels of Death," *Globe and Mail* April 22, 1996, A15.

Spudis, E. V. "The Persistent Vegetative State," *Journal of Neurological Sciences*, 102 (1991): 128-36.

Notes

1 E. Becker, *The Denial of Death* (New York: Free Press, 1973).
2 All scriptural quotations in this article are taken from the New International version of the Bible, copyright the New York International Bible Society.
3 Genuis, S. J., and Genuis, S. K. "Living and Dying with Dignity," *Journal of the Society of Obstetricians and Gynaecologists of Canada* 16, no. 6, (1994): 1771-74.
4 Editor's note: As the state of Oregon has done.
5 Judge Stephen Reinhard, quoted in Henry Weinstein, "Assisted Deaths Ruled Legal," *Los Angeles Times* March 7, 1996, A1.
6 Alasdair MacIntyre, *After Virtue* (Notre Dame, Ind.: University of Notre Dame Press, 1981).
7 Dr. Dan Stevens (Director), Letter to CMDS-US Members, March 1996.
8 Multi-Society Task Force on PVS, "Medical Aspects of the Persistent Vegetative State," *New England Journal of Medicine* 330 (1994): 1499-1508, 1572-79.
9 R. C. Bone and E. C. Rockow, WEGJG, "Ethical and Moral Guidelines of the Initiation, Continuance and Withdrawal of Intensive Care," *Chest* 97 (1990): 949-58.
10 E. V. Spudis, "The Persistent Vegetative State," *Journal of Neurological Sciences* 102 (1991): 128-36.
11 CMDS-US. Passed unanimously by the CMDS House of Delegates, May 3, 1994, Toronto, Canada.

John Senn

Advance Directives for Health Care: A Christian Appraisal

An advance directive for health care is a document which enables a capable person to specify the type of health care desired, and the document takes effect when that person is incapable of making health care decisions. Usually, the directive relates to medical care desired at the time of a terminal illness. The document may have two parts. The instruction directive specifies the types of care desired in various medical circumstances late in the course of terminal illness. The proxy directive, or durable power of attorney for health care, indicates the surrogate who will aid in making medical decisions when the patient is incapable and terminally ill. The advance directive may relate only to life-sustaining treatments, but in some jurisdictions also specifies the type of management desired for nutrition, place of residence, and other health concerns. The document acts as a guide for health care personnel and families, and has legal force in many parts of Canada and the United States.[1]

Background

Over the last several centuries, and especially since the Enlightenment, man has had increasing confidence in the ability to control both his surroundings and his own life. In particular, the application of scientific investigation to man's surroundings and man himself has been exceptionally productive and has led to many beneficial technological advances and increased control of the physical aspects of life. The benefits have increased man's power and confidence in his abilities; recently, however, harms to our surroundings have been evident, leading to widespread ecological concerns. The harm is not limited to the physical environment, but is also manifest in man's distrust of science and authority, leading man to seek alternative sources of meaning and security.

In medicine, increasing ability to effectively treat disease has been remarkable, and many previously fatal disorders are now curable. Many advances in sanitation, housing, surgery, and pharmacology have resulted from technologic achievements, and many persons are living longer and healthier lives. However, it is now clear that the application of many medical, surgical, and pharmacological modalities have harmful as well as beneficial results. Following treatment, some patients may be left with considerable disability and a quality of living that is unacceptable to them, their families, and society. Much of the distrust of medicine is related to the perception of excessive medical treatment, and many patients wish for greater control over the care they receive so as to prevent possible harms. The ethical response to this patient concern has been embodied in the doctrine of informed consent.

Informed consent or choice has three major components:

1. Information regarding a proposed plan of treatment must be disclosed in understandable terms to the patient with adequate discussion of risks, benefits, and alternatives.
2. The patient must understand the information provided and the implications of treatment and non-treatment.
3. The choice to accept or reject the treatment plan must be free of coercion or undue influence.

Informed choice is now a legal requirement, and is an ethical aspect of the patient's self direction. When the doctrine is applied under ideal circumstances, the patient and the medical advisor participate together in making a prudent medical decision consistent with the patient's wishes.[2]

Making health care decisions for the person who is incapable of that act has always been problematic. Decision-making by surrogates has been used for some time. The best proxy decision consistent with the patient's view would be a "substitute judgment" made by a surrogate who would express the treatment wishes of the patient. If the surrogate does not know the patient's desires or values, the "best interest" decision depends on the surrogate's conception of what is appropriate in the situation. Members of the patient's family or loved ones of the patient are favoured over health care providers as surrogates because of their long-standing concern and knowledge of the incapable patient. Over the past three decades, living wills have been used increasingly frequently, and in 1976 legislation established the living will as a legal document in California. Since that time, many jurisdictions in the United States and Canada have legislated and legalized advance directives. In this way governments have attempted to respect the autonomy of incapable patients in relation to their health care wishes.

To appraise advance directives for health care, this paper explores five topics.

1. What are the benefits of advance directives?
2. Are there disadvantages of advance directives?
3. What is the public response to advance directives?
4. Whose life is it, anyway? A Christian reflection on autonomy
5. Suggestions for a Christian advance directive

Benefits of Advance Directives

Advance directives are designed to improve the health care of decisionally incapable persons by honouring previously expressed wishes, minimizing suffering, and avoiding excessive therapy, thus leading to more patient comfort during the treatment of terminal illness. The documents promote this aim in several ways.

The directive extends the autonomy of the patient to a future time when impairment occurs and thus honours the wishes of the patient for certain types of medical care. The document ensures the patient's values are reflected in the last acts of one's life, if one becomes incapable of decision. In terms of justice, the directive tries to extend the rights of the competent person to a future time if the person should become incompetent. In view of the fact that many persons are members of a community with specific values, the advance directive also promotes that community's ethics and opinions. The document therefore helps to insure that the patient's previous wishes and the values of the person's community are followed rather than medical decisions being made by "moral strangers." Carefully constructed directives may aid family, loved ones, and health care personnel to function more effectively by diminishing their anguish, and by promoting more genuine ethical caring for the incompetent patient. Directives also encourage discussion around the topic of dying and death and increase communication and consideration of values by the patient and the proxy.[3]

Harms Associated with Advance Directives

Directives may fail to promote the incapable patient's desires and health interests. Indeed there is philosophic concern that the incompetent patient is a different person from the previously well person who made the advance directive: if this is true the values expressed in the directive may be false for the person now incapable. At the least, the incapable and capable person have morally significant differences, in that the well person is autonomous and the incapable person may no longer be autonomous. If these philosophic suppositions are true, the use of a written form directing the care of a different person is a "moral cop-out" allowing the health care profession, loved ones, and society to have unfounded confidence in treatment decisions.[4]

If one assumes that the incapable patient is still the same person with the same values as were present at the time of making the directive, several factors still make acceptance of the document questionable. The difficulties of accurate prognosis make the determination of terminal illness problematic. There are many ambiguities and uncertainties to be faced by the patient and health care personnel, and the situation frequently changes from day to day. The presence of unforeseen circumstances influencing optimal patient care is a medical reality and calls for the ability to accommodate these changes with new decisions. Provided the instruction directive is general and flexible enough to accommodate changes recommended by the chosen proxy, the aims of the patient may be met. If the proxy is an effective maker of a "substitute decision" on behalf of the patient, appropriate participatory decision making with the health care providers may be in the patient's best interest. Otherwise, the health care provider may be required to follow the written instruction directive, thus abandoning the now incompetent patient to an autonomous choice made at a previous time. The use of vague terms, such as "heroic measures" diminishes the clarity of the directive and further contributes to ambiguity in implementation.[5]

Further concerns relate to the demonstrable instability in patient wishes, especially those of well persons trying to visualize and express their wishes at a time when they become incapable and ill.[6] The training of health care workers to explain and aid persons in making directives is often limited especially if the health care person is not aware of the patient's values and life plan.[7] Concern has also been expressed that advance directives may be used to promote cost savings and rationing for incompetent persons, but evidence against these fears is available.[8]

Acceptance of advance directives may lead to future harms. The definition of "terminal" illness is imprecise, and may be interpreted so broadly that therapy may be withdrawn many months or even years before an estimated time of death. For example, treatment limitation for "terminal" illness may be extended to patients with long-standing incompetence who may live for many months or years. This group of patients is significant in number and includes those in persistent vegetative state, long-standing coma, and progressive dementia. Use of medical directives as a platform to enable euthanasia or physician assisted suicide to occur must be avoided.[9] Persons may also formulate advance directives indicating that they do not wish forms of therapy which may return them to excellent life quality, thus prejudicing curative health care. As well at this stage advance directives permit individuals to limit care, but do not allow demands for certain types of care to be given. Concern has been expressed that directives legalizing demands for medically inappropriate and unnecessary care may be formulated.[10]

Response of the Public to Advance Directives

Extensive medical literature is available indicating the reaction of well persons, patients, health care workers, and society to advance directives. The support of the general public for advance directives has been documented, indicating that 89% were in favour of advance directives, and similarly outpatients who were reasonably healthy favoured advance directives by a large majority (93%).[11] In view of these findings, it is surprising that no more than 10 to 20% of patients entering hospital will undertake the preparation of an advance directive when it is offered to them.[12] The reasons for reluctance to complete the directives are unclear, although reluctance to consider death and end of life matters, or the time required to fill out the document, may be contributory. However, we have done a small study of attitudes of the healthy and unwell to the treatment of terminal illness. Older persons who were healthy and older patients who had terminal illness were asked regarding their wishes for "full care" or "comfort care." Our results suggest that the experience of sickness changes the attitudes to terminal illness, that directives should be reconsidered if the person has prepared the directive in good health and is subsequently diagnosed with terminal illness, and that decisionally impaired persons may not receive the type of care that was indicated in their advance directive.[13] The general acceptance of advance directives by legislators and the law may reflect the fact that the legislators and lawyers making the decisions are healthy rather than terminally ill.

The reluctance of ill persons to fill out advance directives may also relate to selecting a proxy. Difficulties in speaking about dying and a wish not to place undue pressure on a close relative may play a part. There is also considerable evidence that proxy predictions frequently do not meet the requirement of "substituted judgment." The failure of adequate and repeated discussion between the proxy and the competent person often leads to decisions being made which are not consonant with the incapable person's wishes expressed when the person was competent.[14]

Health care workers also have concerns about advance directives. It has been shown that physicians' opinions regarding patient wishes for life sustaining therapy are frequently at variance with patients' desires. Moreover, health care workers are apprehensive that a poorly constructed advance directive or an uninformed proxy may lead to inferior care for an incompetent patient who might recover. The time and effort to discuss and complete an initial advance directive and to be sure that appropriate follow up is done is a considerable demand on the patient, loved ones, and health care personnel.[15]

At this time the legislative and legal acceptability of advance directives is overwhelming. In view of the many problems associated with advance directives it is necessary to carefully construct, discuss, and implement the documents.

Whose Life Is It Anyway? A Christian Reflection on Autonomy

In the past century, the principle of self-direction and control of one's own life has been increasingly accentuated. For instance, a landmark legal decision in 1914 by Justice Benjamin Cardozo stated "Every human being of adult years and sound mind has a right to determine what shall be done with his own body," thus affirming the principle of respect for autonomy.[16] Building on previous philosophical work, many contemporary ethicists have advanced the view that self direction is of cardinal importance in medicine.[17] Others are now suggesting that patient autonomy should be less dominant, and that increased value should be ascribed to other ethical approaches such as justice, the common good, caring, relationships, and virtues. At this time, continuing efforts are needed to balance respect for the patient's autonomy with other ethical and social factors in our diverse and pluralistic society with its changing and multiple beliefs.[18]

Christians have an unique contribution to make in today's ethically diverse milieu,[19] and part of the gift is in the understanding of autonomy in a Christian way. Many of the values associated with the importance of man and the need to respect him are in keeping with Christian beliefs: indeed the idea of man in the image of God (*imago Dei*) and Irenaeus' statement that "Life in man is the glory of God: the life of man is the vision of God" gives some idea of the high regard that Christians have for man.[20] However, the tendency of autonomy to merge with extreme individualism is a secular proclivity, out of keeping with Christian belief.

The Christian understanding of man's importance follows from the belief that God is man's creator, sustainer, and redeemer. "Male and female, they will be like us and resemble us. . . . God created human beings" (Gen 1:26, 27).[21] Created by God, and in the image of God, humans are good and valuable. "The Spirit also comes to help us, weak as we are" (Rom 8:28). God in the person of his Spirit helps and sustains us. "We have placed our hope in the living God, who is the Saviour of all" (1 Tim 4:10). The Christian also believes that Jesus Christ, the Son of God, lived a fully human life and suffered on the Cross for the salvation of man from his sins, making it possible for man to participate in God's Kingdom on earth; and through his death and resurrection to enter God's Kingdom in eternal life. These Christian beliefs give a new comprehension of meaning for human earthly life, and provide new understanding for the nature of Christian self-direction.

. The framework for self-directed choice which follows from Christian belief is in marked contrast to autonomy considered on secular grounds. The secularist regards autonomy as self-directed freedom to control one's own life, to support personal (individual) rights, and to form a bulwark against the aggression of other persons: he demands respect and rights. On the other hand, the Christian regards autonomy as self-directed freedom to choose life "in Christ" and "responsible stewardship" toward God and his creation, including human beings. The belief in the goodness of God's creation and God's concern for human beings compels the Christian to follow the two commandments: "Love the Lord your God with all your heart, with all your soul, and with all your mind. . . . Love your neighbour as you love yourself" (Mt 22:37, 39).

As the person "in Christ" attempts to follow these commandments, he realizes that following Christ, being "in Christ," requires facing the example of Christ on the Cross. The suffering of the crucified Christ is for man and the world, and St. Paul's witness suggests that Christians may help "to complete what still remains of Christ's sufferings" (Col 1:24). Also we are told "The greatest love a person can have for his friends is to give his life for them" (Jn 15:13). These biblical quotations suggest that suffering is a part of life "in Christ," and provide meaning, encouragement, and strength to endure for the Christian who suffers. The attitude and bearing of the Christian is in contrast to the lack of meaning, despair, and reluctance of many secular persons in the presence of suffering.

The Christian values founded on God's revelation and commandments as expressed above influence the Christian's self-directed freedom of choice, and thus contribute to the way in which Christians interpret the question "whose life is it anyway?" Many Christians regard life as a gift given by God to man: the gift has great value, and man's response is to live "in Christ." The gift of life and freedom to choose one's direction leads the Christian to be a responsible steward of life, and to respect the freedom of each person to make his choice. Thus the Christian makes self-directed choices "in Christ" which always express the person's respect for God and his fellow man. To the question "Whose life is it anyway?" the Christian answers "life is God's precious gift to be lived by man's free choice 'in Christ' in participation with his fellows and in caring for God's creation."

Suggestions for Forming an Advance Directive for Christians[22]

First, the Christian understanding of autonomy leads to a form of advance directive that differs significantly from a secular document. In each case the directive reflects a differing concept of the meaning of life, leading to very different interpretations of how one expresses freedom of choice. The underlying concepts are often expressed and formulated vaguely if at all, so that the different choices made may be at variance with true values of the person making the directive. For this reason, the expression of personal values forces clarity of understanding, and construction of the directive is more apt to reflect the person's true wishes. The advance directive made by a Christian should contain a preamble expressing in a general way the person's underlying values, especially those relating to health care in illness.

Second, the directive should express wishes related to the types of care to be provided in terminal illness: in particular the directive should address the use of life sustaining measures and of care designed to improve comfort. Extending wishes for types of care to be provided in non-terminal states (i.e., conditions in which life is expected to persist many months or years) requires special consideration and advice. In no case should the caregiver be expected to provide care with the intent of causing death.

Third, the advance directive should include an instruction and proxy component. Written instructions should be as clear as possible, but remember that inflexible written directions limiting care in terminal illness must be honoured! Vague instructions are often of no use, as interpretations may differ widely. Proxy directives are useful provided that the proxy knows and will interpret faithfully the recently discussed values and wishes of the patient. A proxy providing "substituted judgment" can participate effectively with other loved ones and care providers in honouring the values and wishes of the incompetent person.

Fourth, advance directives should be reviewed regularly, especially with change in health status. Though a person's values alter slowly, the life plans and health care wishes expressing those values may change more frequently.

Fifth, cooperation of patient, proxy, and health care provider is recommended in formulating or completing an advance directive. The patient should know his values and wishes. The proxy should know the values and wishes of the patient, and be trusted to interpret and honour the patient's view. The health care person should explain the medical circumstances and wording, and provide opinion relating to medical matters. In this way, a satisfactory directive should result. Religious, financial, or legal advisors may also contribute.

Sixth, the advance directive should be available at time of need. The proxy, loved ones, and physician should know where the directive is located. A statement regarding the advance directive may be deposited in the patient's purse or wallet.

Seventh, who should make an advance directive? Any adult. In most jurisdictions, a surrogate is identified if an advance directive is not available. The surrogate is usually a family member or loved one. It is advisable at least to designate a surrogate who is familiar with your life plans and values. Persons without family or loved ones should complete an advance directive.

Eighth, what forms are available? Many forms are produced by government, health care persons, lawyers, advocacy groups, or others. Regardless of your selection, be certain that the document contains values, instruction, and proxy components. Also, complete the document with your proxy, and with medical advice, and be sure the directive is regularly reviewed and accessible.

Summary

Advance Directives for Health Care are documents prepared by a person capable of making a health care decision: the document specifies the type of health care desired if the person becomes decisionally incapable. The documents, their advantages and disadvantages are described. A major aim of the directive is to respect the autonomous wishes of the patient. Both Christian and secular opinion wish to honour a person's freedom to choose: however further exploration uncovers important differences in Christian and secular conceptions of self-direction. The differences identified make the expression of values a necessary component in forming an advance directive, especially for the Christian person. This appraisal of advance directives concludes that they are a useful device for assuring that the competent person's values and life plans are honoured if incompetence ensues. Suggestions are proposed for preparing an advance directive for the Christian person.

Notes

1 Advance Directives Seminar Group, Centre for Bioethics, University of Toronto, "Advance Directives: Are They an Advance?" *Canadian Medical Association Journal* 146, no. 2 (1992): 127–34.

2 T. L. Beauchamp and J. F. Childress, *Principles of Biomedical Ethics*, 3rd ed. (New York: Oxford University Press, 1989), 75.

3 Advance Directives Seminar Group, "Advance Directives," 127–34; J. M. McIntyre, "Shepherding the Patient's Right to Self-Determination," editorial in *Archives of Internal Medicine* 152 (1992): 259–61; E. H. Loewy, *Freedom and Community: The Ethics of Interrelationships* (Albany, N.Y.: SUNY Press, 1992).

4 E. H. Loewy, "Advance Directives and Surrogate Laws: Ethical Instruments or Moral Cop-out?" *Archives of Internal Medicine* 152 (1992): 1973–76.

5 Advance Directives Seminar Group, "Advance Directives," 127–34; McIntyre, "Shepherding the Patient's Right," 259–61; C. J. Ryan, "Betting Your Life: An Argument Against Certain Advance Directives," *Journal of Medical Ethics* 22 (1996): 95–99; A. S. Brett, "Limitations of Listing Specific Medical Interventions in Advance Directives?" *Journal of the American Medical Association* 266 (1991): 825–28.

6 M. Danio et al., "Stability of Choices About Life-Sustaining Treatments," *Annals of Internal Medicine* 120 (1994): 567–73.

7 S. M. Wolf et al., "Sources of Concern about the Patient Self-Determination Act," *New England Journal of Medicine* 325, no. 23 (1991): 1666–71.

8 L. J. Schneiderman et al., "Effects of Offering Advance Directives on Medical Treatments and Costs?" *Annals of Internal Medicine* 117 (1992): 599–606.

9 P. L. Jaggard, "Advance Directives: A Case for Greater Dialogue?" in *Bioethics and the Future of Medicine: A Christian Appraisal*, ed. J. F. Kilner, M. N. Cameron, and D. L. Schiedermayer (Grand Rapids, Mich.: Eerdmans, 1995), 250–62.

10 E. D. Pellegrino, "Patient Autonomy and the Physician's Ethics," *Annals of the Royal College of Physicians and Surgeons of Canada* 27 (1994): 171–73.

11 L. L. Emanuel et al., "Advance Directives for Medical Care: A Case for Greater Use?" *New England Journal of Medicine* 324 (1991): 880–95.

12 S. M. Wolf et al., "Sources of Concern," 1666–71.

13 M. C. Tierney et al., "How Reliable are Advance Directives for Health Care? A Study of Attitudes of the Healthy and Unwell to Treatment of the Terminally

Ill," *Annals of the Royal College of Physicians and Surgeons of Canada* 25, no. 5 (1992): 267–70.

[14] N. R. Zweibel and C. Cassell, "Treatment Choices at the End of Life: A Comparison of Decisions by Older Patients and Their Physician-Selected Proxies," *The Gerontologist* 29, no. 5 (1989): 615-21; J. Hare et al., "Agreement Between Patients and Their Self-selected Surrogates on Difficult Medical Decisions," *Archives of Internal Medicine* 152 (1992): 1049-54; A. B. Seckler et al., "Substituted Judgment: How Accurate are Proxy Predictions?" *Annals of Internal Medicine* 115, no. 2 (1991): 92-98; M. A. Lee and K. Berry, "Abuse of Durable Power of Attorney for Health Care: Case Report," *Journal of the American Geriatric Society* 39 (1991): 806-9.

[15] B. Lo et al., "Patient Attitudes to Discussing Life-Sustaining Treatment," *Archives of Internal Medicine* 146 (1986): 1613-15; M. Danis et al., "A Prospective Study of Advance Directives for Life-Sustaining Care?" *New England Journal of Medicine* 324 (1991): 882-88; M. Kelner et al., "Advance Directives: The Views Of Health Care Professionals?" *Canadian Medical Association Journal* 148, no. 8 (1993): 1331-38.

[16] *Schloendorff v. New York Hospital*, 211 NY 125, 127, 129; 105 NE, 92, 93 (1914).

[17] H. T. Engelhardt, *The Foundations of Bioethics* (New York: Oxford University Press, 1986), 85ff.

[18] Beauchamp, *Principles of Biomedical Ethics*, 75ff; Loewy, *Freedom and Community*; Jaggard, "Advance Directives," 250-262.

[19] G. Grisez et al., "Practical Principles, Moral Truth, and Ultimate Ends," *American Journal of Jurisprudence* 32 (1987): 99-151; J. S. Horner, "Christian Ethics: An Irrelevance or the Salvation of Medicine?" *Journal of Medical Ethics* 20 (1994): 133-34.

[20] St. Irenaeus, *Treatise against Heresies in Liturgy of the Hours*, 3:1498.

[21] All scriptural quotations in this article are taken from Today's English Version of the Bible, copyright the American Bible Society.

[22] J. DeBlois et al., "Advance Directives of Health Care Decisions: A Christian Perspective," *Health Progress* (July/August 1991): 27-31; Pennsylvania Bishops, "Living Will and Proxy for Health Care Decisions," *Origins CNS Documentary Service* 23, no. 10 (1993): 162-64; W. F. Carr, "Living Wills and Religious Communities," *Linacre Quarterly* 60, no. 2 (1993): 72-77; M. A. Grodin, "Religious Advance Directives: The Convergence of Law, Religion, Medicine and Public Health," *American Journal of Public Health* 83, no. 6 (1993): 899-903.

Stephen Genuis

Reproductive Services: The Need for Ongoing Evaluation[†]

Over the last few decades, the numbers of North American couples experiencing infertility have escalated at the same time as the supply of adoptable newborns has dramatically decreased. The result has been the emergence of a vast array of assisted reproductive technologies (ARTs), many of which raise ethical and legal questions[1] both for individuals and for society.

While assisting couples to realise their dream and become parents is both valuable and personally rewarding, the experimental nature of many ARTs is well recognized both in the medical literature[2] and more recently by the Canadian Government.[3] The very newness of these rapidly proliferating therapies highlights the fact that "sufficient time has not elapsed to permit evaluation of the long-term outcomes for participants and society."[4] Because reproductive technologies may challenge fundamental assumptions relating to parentage, personhood, and even the beginnings of life, thus potentially creating a myriad practical, legal, and ethical dilemmas, it is well recognized that formal guidelines for monitoring and perhaps limiting ARTs need to be developed.[5]

In the past, treatments related to infertility evoked limited interest for those not directly involved, however, the evolution of more controversial technologies and the increase in sensational legal cases have brought the sub-specialty of reproductive medicine into public focus. As research, development, and use of ARTs raise social and

---

[†] Reprint of Stephen J. Genuis and Shelagh K. Genuis, "Reproductive Services: The Need for Ongoing Evaluation," Journal SOGC 17, no. 5 (1995): 481–86. Used by permission.

economic as well as ethical and legal concerns,[6] it is important that the public be both informed and consulted regarding these technologies.

In 1990, an Angus Reid survey found that although Canadians were aware of ARTs, their basic knowledge regarding techniques and procedures was poor. This survey pointed out that most Canadians "have not yet begun to consider many of the long term implications associated with the use of some of these technologies."[7] Although the Royal Commission on New Reproductive Technologies certainly served to increase public awareness in the early 1990s, public attention continues to be focused on the more sensational aspects of ARTs (for example surrogate or post-menopausal child-bearing), while other areas including donor insemination are rarely discussed.[8] In addition, the ever-changing nature of research and technology in this area makes it difficult for lay people and even for physicians to keep pace with recent developments.

In order to assess attitudes towards various ARTs, a public attitude survey was carried out in Western Canada. Using case vignettes as well as general questions, respondents were asked to express opinions about specific ARTs and related issues. Demographic information was also solicited. The survey generated a large data base on a variety of both commonly accepted and more controversial ARTs.[9]

In this paper, findings from the Canadian survey will be highlighted as the issue of gamete donation is reviewed. Despite the familiarity with this infertility therapy, particularly with donor insemination, the increasing number of ethical complexities and the lack of standardized practice illustrate that even the more common ARTs need to be re-examined and guidelines for practice implemented.

Gamete Donation

Therapeutic donor insemination (TDI) has become a commonplace intervention for many infertile couples who are diagnosed with male infertility. This practice has not been without debate, however, for as early as in 1951 this therapy was criticized for its possible negative effects on the relationship between child and legal, though non-genetic father.[10] Although sperm donation has been a relatively accepted practice by many practitioners for some time now, increasing understanding of and interest in issues related to psychological identity and genetic hereditary, the more recent possibilities of egg and embryo donation, and the judicial focus on "best interests" of the child demand that even this well established reproductive service be re-visited and re-evaluated.

As gamete donation has become a more socially accepted practice, increased interest and more detailed public discussion have been facilitated. National public attitude surveys in the area of ARTs have been carried out in Australia and the United Kingdom[11] as well as some smaller surveys examining single aspects of ARTs.[12] In Australia, support for the donation of sperm or eggs received respectively 55% and 56% approval, while both the donation of fertilized eggs and the freezing of embryos received 45% support.[13] A smaller attitude survey of infertile couples who were already pursuing gamete donation indicated a high acceptance of using a sister for ovum donation; in fact 61% of participants had secured such an agreement. In contrast, only 11% of couples undergoing TDI expressed a preference for using a brother as a donor.[14] Another survey, which examined how couples viewed a variety of infertility therapies, found that interventions which produced a child who was "biologically related to only one member of the couple were viewed most negatively."[15]

These findings contrast with some of the attitudes found in the Canadian population. When asked for an answer regarding their willingness to donate gametes to infertile siblings, close friends, or strangers, men and women responded similarly with a marked preference for sibling versus stranger donation[16] (See Table 1). While few (12%) thought that gamete donors should have any legal rights or responsibilities for a resulting child, the majority (59%) indicated that offspring, upon reaching an appropriated age, should have access to information regarding their biological donor parent.[17] These findings concur in part with an Australian survey which found that 90% of participants felt that sperm donors should not have responsibility for resulting children; however, in contrast, 66% of the Aus-

	Egg Donation to			Sperm Donation to		
	Sister	Friend	Stranger	Sister	Friend	Stranger
Overall Support %	66%	49%	41%	63%	49%	44%

TABLE I: Support for gamete donation.

tralian participants felt that the child should not have access to information regarding the donor.[18]

Although gamete donation may appear to be one of the more innocuous reproductive services, there are many related issues which require careful consideration. Potential sources of gametes or embryos, disclosure of biological origins and the "best interest" of the child, and potential responsibility or effect on donors will be explored, in order to illustrate some of the issues that need to be brought into discussion about ARTs.

Source of Gametes or Embryos

Insemination with donor sperm has been practised in various forms for thousands of years. Laws in the Old Testament decreed that a widow without a son was to marry and be impregnated by a brother of her deceased husband in order to conceive a son who would then carry on her first husband's name.[19] Although such insemination was not carried out artificially, the discovery in our age that sperm can be cryo-preserved has greatly enhanced the therapeutic use of donor insemination. There is less acceptance of TDI in some cultural and religious groups[20] but nevertheless, the relatively simple retrieval of male gametes and the development of sperm banking have, for the most part, ensured the availability of sperm for the treatment of male infertility.

Although many in the Canadian survey favoured directed donation of sperm to a known recipient,[21] there are also reports that many favour the more usual practice of anonymous donation.[22] Donor anonymity has, however, been accompanied by a generalized lack of consistent record keeping; in many cases, records of donor medical history have not been maintained and in some clinics it is even difficult to determine how many offspring have been born from a single individual's sperm.[23] This latter issue is particularly important for certain minority groups in smaller centres where the availability of donors may be limited,[24] and consanguinity may be a concern.[25]

Acquiring ova for donation is an invasive process with potential risks to the donor.[26] The acceptability of using a sister for gamete donation has found high approval in a number of studies,[27] and it has been suggested that sibling donors would minimize biological variance, allow easy access to family and medical history, and assist participants to define relationships prior to the child's birth.[28] Conversely, fear has been expressed that in addition to the medical risks sustained by an egg donor, designated donation of eggs could potentially cause difficulty in the child/parent relationship, exploitation of the donor,[29] and conflict between genetic and birth mothers who are known to one another. The Canadian Royal Commission recommended that designated donation of ova be disallowed; yet other authors point out that concerns related to child/parent relationships have not ruled out the practice of intrafamily adoption, nor have concerns of exploitation eliminated the donation of other types of tissue to a designated needy relative.[30]

The acknowledged shortage of eggs for donation gives rise to the concern that coercion may be used on less wealthy, infertile women who themselves wish to undergo egg retrieval for the often costly process of in vitro fertilization (IVP). The possible proposal to donate excess oocytes in exchange for covering the costs of their own reproductive services puts indigent women in a vulnerable position and is clearly equivalent to the selling of gametes, a practice generally condemned.[31] It has also been noted in the medical literature that fetal ovaries, which contain large numbers of immature oocytes, "could be used for in-vitro fertilization or transplantation as a treatment for female infertility;"[32] this practice could potentially be used to circumvent the difficulty in finding donors and to overcome the shortage of oocytes available for donation. At a recent meeting of the American Fertility Society, the use of fetal ovarian tissue was brought into focus by a discussion of collaborative research being carried out between universities in the United States and China. Ovaries from female fetuses, selectively terminated during the second and third trimesters, are reportedly being investigated using a process of induced maturation, fertilization, and potential embryo transfer.[33] This research introduces the possibility that a female fetus who has been aborted may become the biological "mother" of living children. The use of oocytes originating from fetuses raises significant ethical concerns and was recently strongly rejected by the Canadian Royal Commission which recommended that such activity be "prohibited outright in the Criminal Code of Canada."[34] Although not specifically addressing the use of fetal oocytes, Australia's Infertility Act, one of the most comprehensive attempts at regulation in the world, restricts research on embryos and bans the use of children's gametes.[35]

Securing a supply of oocytes for donation is further complicated by the fact that cryo-preservation of these gametes has been largely unsuccessful[36] and the use of fresh ova is not recommended.[37] With the increasing prevalence of human immunodeficiency virus (HIV) in reproductive age women,[38] the risks associated with the use of fresh gametes are clearly recognized.[39] In response to this concern, oocytes are frequently fertilized first and then the resulting zygote is frozen for future use.[40] It is, however, not uncommon for multiple embryos to be produced during the process of IVF and it is possible that couples may wish to donate excess embryos subsequent to their IVF treatment. This type of donation has been compared to adoption,[41] and is seen by many as a positive alternative to the ethical dilemma created by the existence of excess embryos retained in a cryo-preserved state.

Disclosure and Children's "Best Interest"

In recent court cases, debatable parentage has increasingly been judged by the somewhat subjective standard of the child's "best interest." A review of a number of landmark cases and United States Supreme Court decisions indicates that "the Justices considered the best interests of the child and the unity of the family to be paramount."[42] This principle being established, it must be acknowledged that long-term empirical data defining what constitutes "best interest" are frequently unavailable due to the relatively recent explosion in available technologies. For couples who have conceived a pregnancy through gamete donation, one of the most significant decisions which must be faced is whether or not to tell the child about his or her biological background.[43]

While many professionals think that, as in adoption, non-disclosure has tremendous potential for harm and they address the negative effects of that deception on children, parents, and extended family,[44] others argue that the couple has a right not to disclose the use of a donor to the child. Religious and cultural considerations may play a role in the decision for non-disclosure or the couple may feel emotionally unequipped to deal with the child's potential reaction. In the case of anonymous donation, the inability to provide children with information beyond medical history and the possibility that they may have negative feelings about their biological origins may lead couples to question whether revealing the existence of a donor patient would serve the "best interests" of their child.[45]

An additional dilemma with disclosure is that "the appropriate age to tell a child has not been determined."[46] A very young child's inability to choose the appropriate person with whom to share personal information may cause discomfort for that individual at an older age; on the other hand, parents who choose to disclose in later years "fear the child may feel like a 'bomb' has been dropped."[47]

Despite the complications which may be caused by disclosing biological origins, the majority of respondents in the Canadian attitudes survey felt that at an appropriate age, offspring should have access to information about a donor parent.[48] The definite preference for gamete donation to a sibling as opposed to a stranger found in the same survey, suggests that adults who are theoretically considering donation, value genetic linkage over anonymity. The Canadian Royal Commission, however, found that women and couples contemplating TDI preferred an anonymous donor. Recognizing that anonymity may work against the interests of children, the Commission recommended that a registry of non-identifying information should be made available to parents and their TDI offspring.[49]

In jurisdictions where there is legislation regarding TDI, anonymity of the donor is usually protected while giving offspring access to non-identifying information. The exception to this is in Sweden where TDI children have the option upon reaching the age of majority to request a meeting with their genetic parents. The donor gives consent to this meeting prior to donation.[50]

Although analogies can be made to some adopted children who experience a sense of "genealogical bewilderment," little is known about the effect on a child's sense of identity and belonging when they are born from a donated gamete.[51] Some, no doubt, will feel an immense need to know something of their roots. As a very articulate 19-year-old stated in a recent editorial, "I'm a person created by donor insemination, someone who will never know half of her identity. I feel anger and confusion and I'm filled with questions . . . children are not commodities or possessions. They are people with an equal stake in the process."[52]

Long Term Considerations

A large majority of respondents to the Canadian survey (88%) felt that gamete donors should not have any legal rights to, or responsibilities for, a resulting child.[53] This viewpoint reflects the *status quo* as, for the most part, it is assumed that a woman giving birth is the genetic mother and her husband is, at the very least, the responsible father.[54] In the case of gamete donation, however, there is a very real possibility that rights and responsibility may become divisive issues, as only three regions in Canada (Newfoundland, Quebec, and the Yukon Territories) and about half of the American states have enacted legislation to define the status of those involved in TDI and their offspring.[55]

There is a very clear need for further study and legislation to define and protect the rights and responsibilities of parties involved in gamete donation. In areas where family law has not been amended, the possibilities remain that a recipient's spouse may disavow parentage and support for a child, that a recipient may attempt to deny visitation privileges to a spouse following marriage break-up, that a donor may seek to establish parentage, or that recipients and children might seek support or inheritance rights from a donor.[56] Because egg donation is relatively new and still uncommon, judicial rulings and subsequent laws have focused on TDI and questions relating to paternity. Where there has been consent to TDI, courts have "treat[ed] parenthood as a social, rather than a biological phenomenon"[57] thus "surpassing the right of the purely biological/genetic father."[58]

As is eloquently foreshadowed by the personal anguish of some women who have relinquished children for adoption, human reproduction, even simplified to the basic component of gamete donation, may have lifelong implications. The Canadian Royal Commission noted that many sperm donors reported a very casual attitude towards donation until they were married or had their own children; then "they began considering the implications of having a genetically linked child growing up elsewhere."[59] Some donors "strongly regretted" donating, while others reported that their "wives or partners were upset by their past donations."[60]

The long-term effects of participating in gamete donation are largely left to speculation.[61] For a woman who has donated excess eggs while undergoing fertility treatments, there is a chance that a donated egg may gestate successfully while she remains childless. This possibility, even if the donor is unaware of the status of donated eggs, "could cause psychological distress."[62] On the other hand, it has been suggested that couples who are the recipients of egg donation may experience fewer negative feelings than those using a sperm donor. Being able to carry the child, "may mitigate the woman's feeling that she is on the periphery of the pregnancy, as some men may feel when donor sperm is used."[63]

Conclusion

The rapid proliferation of various reproductive therapies has resulted in the ready acceptance of some types of technology "without proper legal, ethical, or moral evaluation to cover the complexities of the resulting product."[64] Even in the case of relatively common, less complicated reproductive services, such as gamete donation, there are still important unresolved legal and ethical questions. Once such a medical procedure is established and readily available, ongoing evaluation in light of new research findings and legal reality becomes even more challenging.

Although there is a definite need for legally enacted guidelines in the area of reproductive services, the medical community also has a responsibility to "have an impact on society by providing policies that ensure accountability."[65] Expanding medical technology, interacting with changing social needs and increasing legal complexity, demands that standards of practice be established with an inherent mechanism for re-evaluation on an ongoing basis.

Notes

[1] M. V. Sauer et al., "Survey of Attitudes Regarding the Siblings for Gamete Donation," *Fertil Steril* 49 (1988): 721-22; C. Levine., ed., *Taking Sides, Clashing Views on Controversial Bioethical Issues*, 2nd ed. (Guilford, Conn.: Dushkin, 1987).

[2] Ethics Committee of the American Fertility Society, "Ethical Considerations of the New Reproductive Technologies," *Fertil Steril* 53, supp. 2 (1990): 6; S. A. Garcia, "Reproductive Technology for Procreation, Experimentation, and Profit," *J Legal Med* 11 (1990): 1-57; A. M. Braverman and M. E. English, "Creating Brave New Families with Advanced Reproductive Technologies," NAACOGS *Clinical Issues in Prenatal and Women's Health Nursing* 3 (1992): 353–

63.

3   Royal Commission on New Reproductive Technologies, *Proceed with Care; Final Report of the Royal Commission on New Reproductive Technologies* (Ottawa: Canada Communications Groups, 1993).

4   Braverman.

5   Royal Commission; E. E. Wallach, "Medicolegal and Ethical Problems of Assisted Conception," *Current Opin Obstet Gynecol* 2 (1990): 726–31.

6   Royal Commission.

7   D. Vienneau, "Few Favor Government Funding for Test-tube Babies, Studies Shows," *Toronto Star* October 16, 1990, D1.

8   R. Rowland, and C. Ruffin, "Community Attitudes to Artificial Insemination by Husband or Donor, In Vitro Fertilization, and Adoption," *Reprod Fertil* 2 (1983): 195–206.

9   S. J. Genuis, W. C. Chang, and S. K. Genuis, "Public Attitudes in Edmonton Toward Assisted Reproductive Technology," *Can Med Assoc J* 149 (1993): 153–61.

10 H. D. Larnsen, W. J. Pinard, and S. R. Meaker, "Sociologic and Psychological Aspects of Artificial Insemination and Donor Sperm," *JAMA* 13 (1951): 1062–64.

11 G. T. Kovacs, G. M. Wood and M. Brumby, "The Attitudes of the Australian Community to Treatment of Infertility by In Vitro Fertilization and Associated Procedures," *J In Vitro Fertil Embryo Transfer* 2 (1985): 213–16; Morgan Research Centre (Australian affiliate of Gallup International): British Survey conducted Sept. 22–27, 1982.

12 Sauer; Rowland; R. Lessor et al., "A Survey of Public Attitudes Toward Oocyte Donation Between Sisters," *Hum Reprod* 5 (1990): 889–92.

13 Kovacs.

14 Sauer.

15 L. J. Halman, A. Abby, and F. M. Andrews, "Attitudes About Infertility Interventions Among Fertile and Infertile Couples," *Am J Public Health* 82 (1992): 191–94.

16 Genuis.

17 Ibid.

18 Rowland.

19 Deut 25:5-6 (NIV).

20 J. G. Schenker, "Religious Views Regarding Treatment of Infertility by Assisted Reproductive Technologies," *J Assist Reprod Genetics* 9 (1992): 3–8.

21 Genuis.

22 Royal Commission.

23 Ibid.

24 Schenker.

25 Royal Commission.

26 Ibid.

27 Sauer; Genuis.

28 Sauer et al.; Braverman et al.; Royal Commission.

29 Royal Commission.

30 D. Riegar, "Gamete Donation: An Opinion on the Recommendations of the Royal Commission on New Reproductive Technologies," *Can Med Assoc J* 151 (1994): 1433–35.

31 Royal Commission.

32 A. Fine, "Transplantation of Fetal Cells and Tissue: An Overview," *Can Med Assoc J* 151 (1994): 1261–68.

33 L. Little, "Fetal Tissue May Be New Oocyte Supply," *Med Post* 30 (1994): 24–25.

34 Royal Commission.

35 Garcia.

36 Ibid.

37 E-HW Kluge and C. Lucock, *New Human Reproductive Technologies, A Preliminary Perspective of the Canadian Medical Association* (Ottawa: Canadian Medical Association, 1991).

38 P. J. J. Boyer, "HIV Infection in Pregnancy," *Pediatric Ann* 22 (1993): 406–12; D. L. Church and M. J. Gill, "Human Immunodeficiency Virus Infection in Women," *Can J Ob/Gyn Women's Health Care* 6 (1994): 611–14.

39 Royal Commission; Kluge.

40 Garcia.

41 Braverman.

42 E. J. Kermani, "Issues of Child Custody and Our Moral Values in the Era of New Medical Technology," *J Am Acad Child Adolesc Psychiatry* 31 (1992): 533–38.

43 Braverman.

44 A. Baran, and R. Pannor, *Lethal Secrets* (New York: Warner Books, 1989).

45 Braverman.

46 Ibid.

47 Ibid.

48 Genuis.

49 Royal Commission.

50 Ibid.

51 Ibid.

52 M. R. Brown, "Whose Eyes are These, Whose Nose?" *Newsweek* March 7, 1994, 123 (10), 12.

53 Genuis.

54 Garcia.

55 Royal Commission.

56 Garcia; Royal Commission.

57 Garcia.

58 Kermani.

59 Royal Commission.

60 Ibid.

61 Braverman.

62 Royal Commission.

63 Braverman.

64 W. S. Keifer, "Preparing for Obstetrics in the Twenty-first Century: Quo Vadis? [Presidential address]" *Am J Obstet Gynecol* 168 (1993): 1787–90.

65 J. E. Tyson, "Moral and Ethical Issues in Reproductive Medicine: A Crisis of Conscience," *Current Opin Obstet Gynecol* 2 (1990): 869–76.

John Patrick

The Beatitudes as a Basis for Christian Ethics

> The absolute worst way to respond to the challenge of secularism is to adapt to secular standards in language, thought and way of life. If members of a secularist society turn to religion at all, they do so because they are looking for something other than that which that culture provides. —Wolfhart Pannenberg[1]

E arly in the first century of the Christian story the different behaviour of Christians from pagans was apparent to the pagan world. The difference was both troubling and attractive to thoughtful observers. Luke reports that the early Christians found "favour with all the people" (Acts 2:47 KJV) but others were concerned that they threatened the social fabric of the times.

One famous example is of a Roman governor, who wrote to Rome, asking what he should do about these Christians who not only did not commit infanticide on their own children but rescued the exposed children of others. He understood that this different understanding of the sanctity of life would lead to an ever-increasing influence with each succeeding generation. He was correct. But the point which I wish to emphasize is that these changes in behaviour occurred without formal ethical training. My thesis is that a vibrant Christian society will produce "communities of character" to use Stanley Hauerwas' phrase,[2] and I want to talk about two strands of this process.

The Importance of Character
Jesus made it plain to his disciples that they should be different from the pagans around them (Mt 5:46-48, 6:7-8). You must not be like

the heathen, be different and the difference is not merely intellectual; it is to be a question of actions—of character. One can only try to imagine the disciple's response to being told that they were to be the salt of the earth. They undoubtedly picked up the metaphor of preservation much faster than we do but they could be forgiven for wondering how it could be true that they would be the preservative for society. Nevertheless it was.

Today, by contrast, we have papers in the medical literature describing how students are to model empathy without personal involvement. The dominant model for the teaching of medicine, the bio-psycho-social model, is barbarian in its philosophy because it denies the real history of medicine and the spiritual realities of human existence. This denial is carried over into the evaluation of students on the basis of attitudes rather than character because the social scientists say that they can measure attitudes but not character. Thus the history of the Western world, where story and character have been so formative, is dismissed.

Character is the word for what can be expected from individuals or even from nations. The current horror of stereotyping would make us all lonely individuals yet the evidence is that we rapidly form ourselves into groups especially when we are divorced from our formative culture and the language of the heart. Although we are individually responsible for our choices it is the height of arrogance to pretend that our parents, families, churches, schools, and countries do not play a part in who we are.

Most of the trust which is so essential to societal function is based on choices which have been made for us and which we do not usually think about or question until we meet another culture with a different set of givens.

Medical Ethics to Bioethics

I am indebted to the work of Nigel M. de S. Cameron[3] for the insight described in this section. I was aware of how empty were the pontifications of most bioethicists but did not understand why. Dr. Cameron explained the conundrum. Bioethicists are concerned primarily with process and with professionalizing their expertise. Thus, as with most academic activities, certain methodologies are used to divide the *cognescenti* from the hoi polloi. A specialized vocabulary has been developed, and physicians have no necessary part in the conversation. This would be acceptable if the products were arcane but useful. They are not. The medical ethics of the past were in error insofar as they were often reduced to etiquette—but modern bioethics has become so remote from clinical reality as to be equivalent to the activities of medieval schoolmen, except that the consequences of the modern activities can be devastating. When Peter Singer says that a tadpole has more right to exist than a human foetus because the tadpole at least knows which direction it is headed it would be merely fatuous if he thereby lost all influence; but that is not the case.

How Can We Be Good?

Before we get to a specifically Christian understanding of a community of character, I want to say something about other cultures. Students today are even more sensitive about this issue than they were in the past. To most of them it is an article of faith that all cultural opinions are equal—so it behooves us to deal with this question. Wise thinkers in many cultures have struggled with the problem of how the good society is to be nurtured. Socrates was executed for his efforts. This is therefore a subject, which if pursued seriously, is liable to get the teacher into trouble. It is essential to start this discussion with a clear recognition that good pagans made incredible progress in understanding the nature of the good society and they came to formulate very similar codes of ethics. The appendix to *The Abolition of Man*[4] is an easy place to find some of the basic evidence. I take it that this agreement is a reflection of the doctrine that we are all made in the image of God. However, recognizing what is good is only step one. Evil soon rears its ugly head.

The tacit model for understanding evil in the Western world is an educational model, which assumes that the problem of evil is one of ignorance. Goodness is then a problem for educators. Only a moment of serious contemplation is necessary to destroy this naive model. The experience of C. S. Lewis is paradigmatic. After his reluctant acceptance of the truth that God exists, he describes his own first serious thoughts about the reality of creatureliness thus:

> For the first time I examined myself with a serious practical purpose. And there I found what appalled me; a

zoo of lusts, a bedlam of ambitions, a nursery of fears, a
harem of fondled hatreds. My name was legion.[5]

Saint Paul puts it theologically in Romans 7:14-25, where he describes the universal experience of knowing what is good and evil
but being unable to live in coherence with that knowledge. The fact
that no-one claims to be perfect is evidence of the universality of this
phenomenon.

Thus the serious Christian who has faced this reality is committed to a fairly sceptical view of the likely outcome of adult education
in goodness. Courses in ethics make ethicists, not good people.
What thinkers produce is schemes, dreams, and stratagems but
whence cometh the goodness which is found throughout the world;
the goodness that often goes beyond intellectual recognition to practical activity? Furthermore how is it that some societies are more
successful than others and some societies lose their way?

Societal Differences

Although it is a totally unacceptable thought to most of our chatter-
ing classes who pontificate on television, some societies do a better
job than others. For example, tribal warfare in northwestern Europe
during the early centuries after Christ was extremely brutal, and the
treatment of women barbaric. The Babylonians were similarly for-
midable barbarous foes. Here is Habakkuk's description.

That ruthless and impetuous people, who sweep across
the whole earth to seize dwelling places not their own.
They are a feared and dreaded people, they are a law to
themselves and promote their own honour. . . . They fly
like a vulture swooping to devour; they all come bent
on violence . . . guilty men whose own strength is their
God (Hab 1:6-11).[6]

Similarly the ethical ideas of the Ik did not compare with those
of the Greeks and neither did their behaviour. Colin Turnbull described his own emotions whilst studying the Ik like this:

In what follows there will be much to shock, and the
reader will be tempted to say "how primitive . . . how
savage . . . how disgusting" and above all "how inhuman." In living the experience I said all those things
over and over again. . . . The latter judgement, "how

inhuman" . . . supposes that there are certain standards common to all humanity, certain values inherent in humanity itself, from which the people in this book seem to depart in a most drastic manner. In living the experience, however . . . one finds that it is oneself one is looking at and questioning; it is a voyage in quest of the basic human and a discovery of his potential for inhumanity, a potential that lies within us all.

Most of us are unlikely to admit readily that we can sink as low as the Ik, but many of us do, and with far less cause. I am grateful for my involvement in [this story] . . . it has added to my respect for humanity and my hope that we who have been civilized into such empty beliefs as the essential beauty and goodness of humanity may discover ourselves before it is too late.[7]

Two Paradigms of Virtue: The Inhabited Story and the Renewed Mind

The Jews have survived a most horrendous history, whilst the Hittites, Amorites, and Perrizites have not. Some of the Jewish sages suggest a most remarkable reason for this anomaly. They say it is due to taking Deuteronomy 6 seriously. Now in the short space available to me I can only sketch the outline of their wise insights. The story goes like this. Moses warned the Children of Israel that whilst the rigour of the desert life had kept them close to God, numerous lapses notwithstanding, the promised land would be a different story. In effect Moses says, "Houses you did not build, vineyards you did not plant, and cisterns you did not dig" come with a divine warning because they are dangerous to your metaphysical health. Even the overwhelming experience of God at Sinai did not prevent wrong choices and make the Children of Israel good. They broke the first three commandments almost instantly. Moses does, however, offer some guidance. The law of the Lord must be taught to your children diligently, in ordinary conversation at your dining room table, and when your son asks you the meaning of all these things you are to tell him the story of God's dealing with the Children of Israel starting with the redemption story. "We were slaves in Egypt under Pharaoh and God brought us out . . . " I believe that what happens when we gossip the story of God's dealings with man at our dining room table is that character is formed. Children learn by modelling, and the biblical story gives them both heroes and anti-heroes, models of courageous and cowardly living. These stories form the grist for the mill of moral reasoning when it starts up sometime after their childhood. We are all formed by our families, we reflexly follow the patterns of behaviour they taught us. For many aspects of life we will never need to re-examine those reflexes if we were blessed with a good family. This is what I mean by inhabiting a story. Good parents have a responsibility to think about the story they are modelling for their children.

They also need to see that the Bible's stories are known by their children. The ethical standards of the Jews were established in this way.

Going Deeper: The Beatitudes

The Old Testament understanding of the law was to teach us what is good, but in the Sermon on the Mount Jesus teaches us that actions are not enough. He is concerned about our hearts. Paul later expresses this new understanding of the function of the law by saying "the law was a school master to bring us to Christ." Christian ethics—the ethics of the disciple—must go deeper and in addition they must reinforce our wonder at the grace of God (even though grace is not mentioned in the whole sermon).

Intellectual honesty is the root of Christian character and Christian ethics. "Blessed are the poor in spirit." Genuine poverty of spirit is produced by being ruthlessly honest about the real state of our souls as Lewis was when he discovered that he was dominated by lust, ambition, fear, and hatred. This is the humbling experience which Jesus prescribes as the starting point for daily discipleship. Why is it a source of blessing? Because it necessarily takes us to the cross and the atonement of Christ which is the only adequate solution. Thomas à Kempis knew this experience when he wrote: "Whoso knoweth himself is lowly in his own eyes and delighteth not in the praises of men." In our witness we need to remember this statement. When we encourage genuine expression of opinion and proper exploration of reality it always leads towards the kingdom.

But it is not enough. The devils believe and tremble. We need the gift of repentance, which is marked by mourning for sin, an incredibly infrequent experience for most of us. It was the granting of repentance unto life to the household of Cornelius that convinced the Jews that the gospel should extend to the Gentiles. Jesus says that the experience of repentance is necessary for the experience of being comforted by him. We need to be much more in prayer for this experience which will form our character in a way that will inevitably change the world.

Such an experience of the grace of God in forgiveness is the prerequisite to meekness. The word translated "meek" also describes a horse broken in and ready to ride. It is not a synonym of weakness but of power under control and exercised without self awareness. It is the character that Christ exemplified when the people said of him "He speaks with authority and not as the scribes." Part of the ethics of a Christian doctor should be the ethics of unconscious moral authority, which is recognized by others. Such a person does inherit the earth in an entirely non-materialistic way. Mother Theresa could be said to be one of the world's richest women in this sense; for surely she is one of the most loved people on earth.

When our character is formed in this way we shall be hungering and thirsting for ever more draughts of these riches and not only for ourselves but also for others. John Stott points out that there are three types of biblical righteousness;[8] the first is legal, a righteousness obtained by faith (Rom 9:30–10:4)—many evangelical Christians are content to stop here. The second is moral, internal, of the heart (Mt 15:15-20) and is acquired by attention to the mind. Every epistle makes this point. The third is social. The Bible insists that the reality of the first two is demonstrated by the third (Is 1:15-17, 1 Sam 15:22b). To satisfy this thirst we must continue to drink (Jn 4:13) until we are finally satisfied in heaven (Rev 7:16-17). Can you imagine what an impact we would have if instead of being intimidated by political correctness we hungered after righteousness?

We are to be merciful; mercy differs from grace in that it deals with visible pain misery and distress—the results of sin; grace deals with the sin. It is a characteristic of God (Hos 11:8-9) and it is to be characteristic of us too. It is a thousand miles away from empathy because it comes from real involvement in the pain of the sufferer. When Jesus wept at the tomb of Lazarus and lamented over Jerusalem he was showing us the emotional and spiritual cost of real mercy. The test of the Christian is that he shows mercy to all because of his appreciation of the mercy he has received. Paul's claim to be the chief of sinners (1 Tim 1:15) is not, as one might think, a piece of hyperbole but simply the response of a man who knows his own heart so much better than that of anyone else. His response is to pour himself out for the gospel.

What is purity of heart? Psalm 86:11-12 expresses the essential thought: "Unite my heart to fear thy name." The pure in heart are free from the tyranny of the divided self. As with righteousness there is a practical aspect which finds its expression in transparent sincerity, the "single eye" of Matthew 6:22. I like to paraphrase this beatitude as "Blessed are those with no hidden agendas for they shall be removed from all committees." Our world is driven by the desire to have secret knowledge, to be one of the insiders but the disciple is to be a person who lives continuously in God's sight, and God looks upon the heart. The biblical standard of purity is therefore internal and of the heart. The writer to the Hebrews says that this kind of purity is necessary for a confident approach to God (Heb 10:22). Paul is concerned with this idea when he talks about every thought being brought captive to Christ (2 Cor 10:5).

Peacemaking will follow because the major cause of disagreements is lack of openness. James 4, Colossians 1:20, and Ephesians 2:15 show why peacemakers (reconcilers) are the sons of God. But we should be careful to distinguish peace and appeasement. They are very different: to proclaim peace where there is no peace is not Christian (Jer 6:14). Peace demands the pain of apologies, rebukes, and sometimes the refusal to forgive without repentance—cheap peace, like cheap grace, is peace without the cross and without confession. If you think this a minor point, remember that Paul in 2 Corinthians 5:20 beseeches the Corinthians to be reconciled to God; and John, in Revelation 3:20 is asking Christians to open the door of their hearts to Christ!

Persecution is to be expected and taken as a blessing if it is for Christ and for righteousness, and not because we are angular and difficult people. But why joyful? Because of the reward and the purpose, which is to refine our faith (1 Pet 1:6-7), and because it is for him (Lk 6:23).

What emerges from these wonderfully rich words of Jesus is a way of living, a set of ethics, if you will, that transcend anything found elsewhere. Christian ethics flow out of the realities of sin, forgiveness, and hope because Christ died for us and lives within us. We have to work out this wonderful salvation with fear and trembling. The rest of the Sermon on the Mount is a wonderful exposition of how this is to be done, the dangers to be avoided, and the disciplines to be acquired. In the space available to me I can only hope to whet your appetite for Our Lord's instructions on how we ought to live.

From the character formed by the beatitudes Jesus says that he could confidently predict that his disciples would act as salt to preserve the good and light to show the way to God. They would, says Jesus, see our good works and glorify our Father.

The remainder of chapter five deals with a problem that ought always to occupy the minds of Christians thinking about ethics, the problem of shallow legalism. Jesus uses six examples to convict us all of holding too shallow a view of the good. For Jesus it is a matter of the heart. Christians fall from grace most often for three reasons: impurity of thought, self-indulgence, and the neglect of the four guiding duties of Acts 2:42—the apostle's doctrine (reading the Bible), the breaking of bread (the Eucharist), fellowship, and prayers. In chapter six Jesus takes issue with the practice of our faith: our giving, our praying, our fasting, our choice of treasures, our thinking, our service (God or money, freedom is an illusion), and our anxieties. In chapter seven, he focuses on our relationships and particularly the need to avoid wrongful judgment and practise right judgment. In medical schools today to have a judgmental attitude is the most heinous crime, but Jesus is more subtle. He tells us not to judge hypocritically, to wish to remove the splinter from our brother's eye when we have a log in our own. But he does not stop there, he says when you have dealt with your own major problem you can help your brother with the minor problem. Those who have been cured of log disease can help those with splinter disease and there is no risk of pride because step one is to share your own experience of grace and mercy. Jesus then further emphasizes the need for his disciples to judge wisely, to be discreet and sensitive. It is difficult, he says, but apply for divine help and it will be given. He particularly warns us to beware of our teachers. If their lives and their words do not match be exceedingly cautious.

Jesus also says something else which puzzled me greatly for a while. He talks about a broad way which leads to destruction and a narrow way which leads to life. It is traditional to interpret this as the way of the world and the way of the believer, but I think this interpretation is not correct because it would be the only verse in the Sermon which is addressed to unbelievers. I therefore cautiously offer the following suggestion which also happens to describe my own false choices for many years. If Jesus is talking about believers then the broad way would describe those who accept salvation but continue to set their own agendas. That, says Jesus, is dangerous and will be associated with loss. Paul seems to say the same thing in 1 Corinthians 3. The narrow way would then become the way of the cross, "Not my will but thine be done," and that, says Jesus, leads to life, the only truly rewarding life. This interpretation also fits with the final parable. Jesus compares two men who hear his word but only one does his word. To me this is the challenge of the Sermon on the Mount. So many years of my life were passed in undistinguished living that, despite "believing," there would not have been enough evidence to convict me of being a Christian. I have no doubt at all that a deep meditation on the words of Jesus in Matthew 5-7 would transform our lives, and illuminate our ethics. The learning of these three chapters by heart has been the single most important stimulus in my life to increase my desire to be like Jesus. After the riches of the words of Jesus, who would be content with the minimalist sentiments of the Georgetown mantra: justice, autonomy, beneficence, and non-maleficence? "Behold I show you a more excellent way."

Notes

[1] Wolfhart Pannenberg, "How to Think About Secularism," *First Things* 64 (1996): 31.

[2] S. Hauerwas, *A Community of Character* (Notre Dame, Ind.: Notre Dame University Press, 1981).

[3] Nigel M. de S. Cameron, *The New Medicine* (Wheaton, Ill.: Crossway Books, 1991).

[4] C. S. Lewis, *The Abolition of Man* (London: Oxford University Press, 1943).

[5] C. S. Lewis, *Surprised by Joy* (London: Fontana Books, 1959), 181.

6 Unless otherwise noted, all scriptural quotations in this article are taken from the New International version of the Bible, copyright the New York International Bible Society.

7 C. M. Turnbull, *The Mountain People* (New York: Simon and Schuster, Touchstone, 1972), 11-12.

8 John R. W. Stott, *The Message of the Sermon on the Mount* (Leicester, England: Inter-Varsity Press, 1978); for further discussion of the Sermon on the Mount, see M. L. J. Lloyd Jones, *Studies in the Sermon on the Mount* (Leicester, England: Inter-Varsity Press, 1971).

Part III

Virtue of Love

Stanley J. Grenz

Toward a Comprehensive Christian Ethic of Love

Hearing that Jesus had silenced the Sadducees, the Pharisees got together. One of them, an expert in the law, tested him with this question: "Teacher, which is the greatest commandment in the Law?"

Jesus replied, "'Love the Lord your God with all your heart and with all your soul and with all your mind.' This is the first and greatest commandment. And the second is like it: 'Love your neighbour as yourself.' All the Law and the Prophets hang on these two commandments." —Matthew 22:34-40[1]

And now these three remain: faith, hope and love. But the greatest of these is love. —1 Corinthians 13:13

Three months ago, Don and Donna met at a divorced persons' support group. Both had gone through difficult marital break-ups after some twenty years of marriage. These difficulties had seriously wounded the self-esteem of each. In fact, it was these common elements of their stories that initially drew the two together.

One month ago, Don asked Donna to join him for an evening of dinner and dancing. On the dance floor something happened: each found solace in the arms of the other. The last two weeks have been "heavenly" for both. In fact, they have seen each other daily, doing all those "fun" activities together that the day-to-day responsibilities of married life had crowded out of their schedules.

With the increased contact has come increased physical involvement as well. Both Don and Donna are Christians who were raised on the dictum that pre-marital sex is wrong. But both find themselves increasingly desiring to engage in sexual intercourse. As a result, each is struggling in silence with the same question: could it be that the ethic of abstinence is only for adolescents—that the situation is different for mature adults who truly love each other, especially for those who in a previous marriage had known the joys of sex?

◆ ◆ ◆ ◆

George Russell lay in his hospital bed musing about his uncertain future. The prostate surgery had apparently gone without a hitch, thanks to Dr. Jonathan Rogers who was the "best in the business." And in his post-surgical consultation, the specialist had only chuckled when his worrywart of a patient had remarked that the operation had probably not entirely eliminated the problem.

Yet George remained apprehensive. Dr. Rogers had seemed a bit too methodical and matter-of-fact in offering his crisp response to George's expression of anxiety. The patient wished he could feel confident that everything was indeed "going to be all right."

◆ ◆ ◆ ◆

Taking their cue from the conclusion to Paul's great hymn to love (1 Cor 13:13), Christian ethicists have repeatedly extolled the three virtues to which the apostle relegates abiding importance—faith, hope, and love. Traditionally thinkers have termed this trio the "theological virtues," because the distinctive quality of the traits is rooted in the character of God and they are bestowed by God alone.[2]

The great medieval synthesiser of Aristotelian and Christian thought, Thomas Aquinas, spoke of the three as augmenting the four cardinal virtues the Christian tradition inherited from Greece—prudence, courage, temperance, and fortitude. Eight hundred years earlier, however, Augustine offered a narrower focus. Following Paul's conclusion that one of the theological virtues stands above the others, the thinker who is often hailed as the greatest theologian the church has ever produced interpreted the same Greek traits as expressions of the one, central Christian ideal—love.

Our task in this essay is to pursue the course Augustine, like Paul and Jesus before him, charted. Specifically, we want to see in what sense love leads us into the heart of the Christian ethic and determine what characterizes Christian love.

"Love" in the Greek Language

As anyone acquainted with the Christian tradition knows, love is enjoined throughout the Bible. Our Lord did not own the copyright to the answer he gave to the query of the Jewish legal expert (Mt 22:37-40; cf. Mk 12:28-34; Lk 10:25-28). In his response, Jesus summarized the entire Old Testament law as love for God and one's neighbour,[3] a teaching which many of his followers view as—to cite the words of Rudolf Schnackenburg—"the core and climax of the whole of moral doctrine."[4] Although the radical elevation of love may have been unique to Jesus' message,[5] the Teacher himself learned the double command from the Hebrew Scriptures (Deut 6:4-5; Lev 19:18). And as Paul's memorable words to the Corinthian believers indicate (1 Cor 13:13), the apostles passed on the admonition to love they had heard the Master reiterate. What is this quality that we find acclaimed throughout the Bible?

Many scholars have pointed out that in contrast to the impoverished situation of our mother tongue, the language of the New Testament has several words referring to dimensions of what we call "love." If C. S. Lewis is a trustworthy guide, the ancient Greek speaker/writer had available four possibilities: storge (affection, especially within families), philia (friendship), eros (love between the sexes or being in love), and of course agape (charity or self-giving love).[6]

In spite of the array of options that stood before them, the biblical authors were amazingly one-sided in their choice of terms. Two of the four words, storge and eros, did not find their way into the New Testament at all.[7] The third, philia, ranks as the most commonly used term for love in Greek literature. William Barclay describes the richness of the noun and its cognates: "There is a lovely warmth about these words. They mean to look on someone with affectionate regard. They can be used for the love of friendship and for the love of husband and of wife. Philein is best translated to cherish: it includes physical love, but it includes much else beside."[8]

At first glance we might anticipate that the richness of philia would have attracted the attention of the New Testament writers. In fact, however, they use the word only sparingly. The noun itself is found only in James 4:4, where it is put to negative use. In addition, it occasionally appears within related terms, such as philadelphia (e.g., Heb 13:1). The verb phileo is slightly more prominent, occurring about two dozen times (e.g., Mt 10:37). Yet half of these are in the Fourth Gospel, leading Gustav Staehlin to note in the Theological

Dictionary of the New Testament that outside of John "there is no special liking for *phileo*."[9] In short, although *philia* found its way into the canonical writings, the concept did not play the leading role in the thinking of the early church.

In contrast to the relatively meagre presence of the other three terms, the repeated use of *agape* indicates that it is the word of choice in the New Testament. Its prominence leads us to ask, What does this term mean? And how is it related to the other Greek terms for "love"?

Although some observers caution against assuming too strict a demarcation between *agape* and *philia*, a clear distinction does seem to have existed between the two. Staehlin, for example, points out that although in the New Testament *philia* may approach *agape* in meaning, the Greeks sensed a distinction between the two terms similar to our differentiation between "to like" and "to love," especially when accompanied "with strong feeling, inwardness, devotion, and even passion."[10] More significantly, the biblical writers do not generally use *philia* to speak about either God's love for humans or our love for God.[11]

Christians have traditionally drawn an even greater disjunction between *agape* and *eros*.[12] Derived directly from the name of the Greek god who "is compelled by none but compels all," *eros* may be defined as the "passionate love which desires the other for itself."[13] Whether taking the form of sensual intoxication (such as in the fertility rites and temple prostitution of the Greek religious cults) or the more sublime experience of ecstatic union with The One (articulated by Plotinus), the underlying goal was the same. For the Greeks *eros* involved the experience of transcending one's own life.[14]

No wonder Christians from the patristic era into the present have followed the example of the New Testament and elevated *agape* to centre stage.[15] This previously obscure word[16] of uncertain etymology, lacking both the power or magic of *eros* and the warmth of *philia*, was just what the Christians needed to articulate their understanding of love. Why?

In part the answer lies in the meaning of the term itself. In classical Greek, the verb form *agapao* can carry the idea of "to prefer," "to set one good or aim above another," "to esteem one person more highly than another." As a result it could denote God's preference for a particular person and hence the one whom God blesses with particular gifts and possessions. Consequently, *agape* spoke of a love that moved beyond emotion—beyond an experience which, in the words of Barclay, "comes to us unsought, and, in a way, inevitably."[17] Instead, *agape* is "a principle by which we deliberately live."[18] In short, this kind of love has to do with the mind and the will.

In keeping with this distinction, Ethelbert Stauffer draws an illuminating contrast between *agape* and *eros*:

> *Eros* is a general love of the world seeking satisfaction wherever it can. *Agapan* is a love which makes distinctions, choosing and keeping to its object. *Eros* is determined by a more or less indefinite impulsion towards its object. *Agapan* is a free and decisive act determined by its subject. *Eran* in its highest sense is used of the upward impulsion of man, of his love for the divine. *Agapan* relates for the most part to the love of God, to the love of the higher lifting up the lower, elevating the lower above others. *Eros* seeks in others the fulfilment of its own life's hunger. *Agapan* must often be translated "to show love"; it is a giving, active love on the other's behalf.[19]

The Narrative of the Loving God

These distinctions in nomenclature lead us back to the biblical narrative. Indeed, when the writers of Scripture offer ethical teachings, they do not base their statements on an appeal to philology, but to a narrative. Hence, the various dimensions of the biblical ethic arise out of a storyline which focuses on the God who acts in the constancy of divine love.

Forming the backdrop to the story is an affirmation of the universal goodness of God. The biblical writers proclaim the One who sustains all creatures. In love, he provides water, food, and shelter for the animals (Ps 104:10-28) and by his Spirit renews the face of the earth (v. 30). As a loving heavenly Father, God cares for even the most insignificant of creatures—the birds and the grass (Mt 6:26-30).

As important as all creation is, the heart of the narrative lies in a more particular object of divine love. The Bible speaks primarily about God's steadfast, resolute disposition toward humankind. The curtain rises on the drama with the creation of the first humans, followed by the shattering of their bliss through wilful sin. The rest of the story recites how the loving God makes provision for fallen humankind. The Old Testament speaks about God's selection of Abraham to be the one through whom he would bless the nations and God's entering into covenant with Israel. The New Testament, in turn, elevates the story of Jesus as the focal point of God's loving provision and the supreme expression of the divine love. Paul summarizes the biblical narrative in terms of Jesus' self-sacrifice on behalf of miserable human beings: "For you know the grace of our Lord Jesus Christ that though he was rich, yet for your sakes he became poor, so that you through his poverty might become rich" (2 Cor 8:9).

The point is obvious: As we come to see how God has acted toward us—as we understand the biblical narrative—we discover what love truly is. Hence, Paul declares that it was "while we were still sinners" that God demonstrated his love for us by sending Jesus Christ to die (Rom 5:8; cf. 1 Jn 4:10). This grand narrative of the One who freely sacrificed for our sakes led the biblical writers to the previously obscure Greek word *agape*, for this term expressed the self-giving attitude that characterizes the God of the salvation narrative.

The New Testament writers, following the path charted by the Hebrew Scriptures, took the grand biblical narrative one additional step. God's glorious love for us leads us to love also. John stated this truth with sublime simplicity: "We love because he first loved us" (1 Jn 4:19). This love entails a loving response to the One who loved us. Hence, in the early community, Jesus' "first and greatest commandment" quickly became a self-evident assumption (e.g., Jas 1:12; 2:5; 1 Pet 1:8).

This love also quite naturally moves toward others. John, "the apostle of love," summarised the horizontal aspect of the New Testament agapaic ethic in declaring, "since God so loved us, we also ought to love one another" (1 Jn 4:11). The same appeal to the divine narrative is evident in Paul's acknowledgement concerning the Thessalonian believers: "Now about brotherly love we do not need to write you, for you yourselves have been taught by God to love each other" (1 Thess 4:9). Hence, in whatever relational contexts we find ourselves—marriage (Eph 5:22-32), the Christian community (e.g., Rom 14:15), or even a hostile world (1 Pet 2:20-24; 3:9)—believers are to draw from the narrative of the loving God and the self-giving example of Christ the model for living.

Following Jesus' own teaching—"All the law and the prophets hang on these two commandments"—the New Testament writers put forth this agapaic ethic as the fulfilment of the law. In Paul's words, "Let no debt remain outstanding, except the continuing debt to love one another, for he who loves his fellow man has fulfilled the law. The commandments . . . are summed up in this one rule: 'Love your neighbour as yourself'" (Rom 13:8-9; cf. Gal 5:13-14). Hence, *agape* recapitulates the Old Testament law. And by being the bond that unites the individual commandments into a unified whole, love provides the perspective from which believers understand the law.[20]

Why *agape*? Paul seems to offer a threefold answer. In keeping with the ethical teaching of the Old Testament and of Jesus, Paul agrees that love is crucial because it characterizes God. The narrative of God's action on behalf of sinful humankind reveals the greatness of the divine love. As we love, we imitate God.

Further, love lies at the heart of the Pauline ethic because of his assumption that the community of faith is the primary context for living as believers.[21] The Apostle did not conceive of Christ's followers living an isolated, solitary existence, but as called *together* in Christ. Realizing that they form the one body of Christ (e.g., 1 Cor 12:12), believers are naturally to contribute their gifts to the common good (1 Cor 12:5), practise mutuality (Eph 5:21), and evidence Christ-like self-sacrificial concern (Gal 2:2; Phil 2:1-11), even to the point of giving up their personal rights for the sake of others (1 Cor 10:23-33). In a word, community life is the life of love, and *agape* expresses well the idea of life in community.[22] Victor Paul Furnish captures this crucial dimension of the Pauline ethic:

> The believer's life and action are always in, with, and for "the brethren" in Christ. For him, moral action is never a matter of an isolated actor choosing from among a variety of abstract ideals on the basis of how inherently "good" or "evil" each may be. Instead, it is always a matter of choosing and doing what is good for the brother and what will upbuild the whole community of brethren.[23]

The third reason for the agapaic focus is apparent in the climax of Paul's hymn to love.[24] Whereas all other aspects of Christian existence will one day cease, love will carry over into the new aeon. Of the various dimensions of the moral life, therefore, love alone provides insight into the coming age. Indeed, love is the actual quality of the age to come.[25] Hence, for Paul where love exists the new aeon is present. And the moral life is eschatological living: It involves acting now as those who belong to the age to come.

The Foundation for "Agape" in the Divine Life

This discussion of the Pauline focus on *agape* leads us to inquire as to why the narrative of the *loving* God stands at the heart of the biblical drama and thereby forms the foundation for the Christian agapaic ethic. In other words, Why can we say with theological confidence that the God revealed in the biblical narrative is love? The search for an answer to this question leads us into the mystery of the eternal God. Ultimately God's steadfast love for creation, and especially for wayward humankind, arises out of nothing less than the dynamic within the heart of the triune God.

The biblical witness suggests that the God of the salvation narrative is triune, the fellowship of Father, Son, and Holy Spirit. Further, the ontological unity which the three constitute and therefore which comprises the divine essence is *agape*, for as John carefully declared, "God is [as to character or essence] love" (1 Jn 4:8, 16). John's choice of *agape*—the giving of oneself for the other—to describe the divine essential nature is illuminating. As several Christian thinkers as early as Athanasius[26] have noted, the divine unity is comprised by reciprocal self-dedication among the Trinitarian members. God is, therefore, indeed love, for the divine essence is the love that binds together the triune God.

To see this more clearly requires that we set forth an understanding of the dynamic that inheres within the divine life. According to the church fathers, this dynamic involves two movements. Theologians speak of the first movement as "generation." Throughout eternity the Father generates the Son, to use Origen's characterization. This movement does not only constitute the second member of the Trinity who draws his life from the Father. Rather, as Athanasius noted, it also constitutes the first member, for without the Son he is not the Father.[27]

Although differentiated, the Father and the Son are also bound together. The bond between the two is the mutual love they share. Throughout all eternity the Father loves the Son, and the Son reciprocates that love. Augustine noted that the love between the Father and the Son is the Holy Spirit, the eternal Spirit of the relationship[28]—the bond[29]—between the Father and the Son. Being the Spirit of the relationship between the first and second Trinitarian members, the Spirit proceeds from the Father and the Son, according to the Western version of the creed. In this manner, the movement of generation constituting the Father and the Son necessitates as well the procession of the Spirit as the Spirit of the Father and the Son.

God's triune nature as Father, Son, and Spirit indicates how John can truly say "God is love." Love is a relational term, requiring both subject and object (someone loves someone else). Were God a solitary acting subject, God would require the world as the object of his love in order to be the Loving One. But because God is triune, the divine reality already comprehends both love's subject and object—both lover and beloved—as well as the love they share. Consequently, the essence of God does indeed lie in the relationship between the Father and the Son (love), a relationship concretized as the Spirit who is the essence of the one God.

Through all eternity, God is the social Trinity, the community of love. The God who is love cannot but respond to the world in accordance to his own eternal essence—love. Hence, *agape* is not only the description of the eternal God in himself, it is likewise the fundamental characteristic of God in relationship with creation. With profound theological insight, therefore, John bursts forth, "For God so loved the world that he gave . . . " (Jn 3:16).

"Agape" and the Other Dimensions of Love

This theological discussion reminds us that the ultimate foundation for the Christian agapaic ethic resides in the eternal dynamic of the triune God. We fulfil our purpose as those who are to be the *imago Dei* as we love after the manner of God, as our relationships are likewise characterized by *agape*. No wonder Christian ethicists have consistently spoken about the centrality of this kind of love.

But what does the centrality of *agape* say about the related Greek concepts? One solution depicts *agape* as divine love in contrast to *storge, philia,* and *eros* which are merely "natural loves." In his monumental work, *The Four Loves,* C. S. Lewis contrasts the divine "Gift-love" (which God can impart to humans and which in us becomes images of himself) with what he calls the "Need-loves," which "have no resemblance to the Love which God is."[30]

The contrast between *agape* and the other types of love often leads to the elevation of the former over the latter. Paul Tillich, for example, finds the others ambiguous unless they are infused by *agape:* "in the holy community the *agape* quality of love cuts into the *libido, eros,* and *philia* qualities of love and elevates them beyond the ambiguities of their self-centredness."[31] Lewis himself offers a somewhat more optimistic appraisal. He argues that because affection, friendship, and desire are natural loves, *agape* can work through them and thereby bring them to participate in "the eternity of Charity."[32] Lewis writes, "the Divine Love does not *substitute* itself for the natural—as if we had to throw away our silver to make room for the gold. The natural loves are summoned to become modes of Charity while also remaining the natural loves they were."[33]

Lewis's proposal provides an ingenious way through which the human experiences of affection, friendship, and even sexual desire gain access to the transcendent realm of eternity. But his suggestion (even more so than Tillich's[34]) denies that the natural loves enjoy any transcendent grounding, any foundation in the divine life.

Several thinkers today are questioning this traditional focus on *agape.*[35] Given its presence in the New Testament itself, *philia* [friendship] is the obvious choice for rehabilitation. To understand this we must remind ourselves of the classic critique of *philia.* Tillich, following Augustine's lead, articulates the standard appraisal:

> The ambiguities of the *philia* quality of love appeared already in its first description as person-to-person love between equals. However large the group of equals may be, the *philia* quality of love establishes preferential love. Some are preferred, the majority are excluded. . . . *Agape* does not deny the preferential love of the *philia* quality . . . it elevates the preferential love into universal love. . . . *Agape* cuts through the separation of equals and unequals, of sympathy and antipathy, of friendship

and indifference, of desire and disgust. It needs no sympathy in order to love; it loves what it has to reject in terms of *philia*. *Agape* loves in everybody and through everybody love itself.[36]

Recently Gilbert Meilaender has called into question the traditional position exemplified by Tillich. Meilaender wonders if proponents of this view "purchase universal love at the cost (at least in this life) of all particular attachments?" And he points out the dilemma of the pure agapaic ethic: "once we have come to see the goal toward which *philia* calls us, how can we justify continuing to enjoy our preferential loves rather than pressing as best we can toward that goal of universal love even in this life?"[37]

Meilaender's desire to find a place for *philia* within the Christian ethic is laudable in the light of the New Testament use of the cognate word *philadelphia* in injunctions to the Christian community. Hence, Paul admonishes the Romans, "Be devoted to one another in brotherly love" (Rom 12:10; cf. Heb 13:1), although Peter adds the reminder that by itself such love is insufficient (1 Pet 1:22; 2 Pet 1:7). And Paul even uses the cognate verb to speak about our love for Christ, for he warns the Corinthians, "If anyone does not love [*philei*] the Lord—a curse be on him" (1 Cor 16:22).

Even more importantly, the biblical materials suggest that like *agape*, *philia* may find its foundation in the salvation narrative. After speaking about the great love that would lead him to lay down his life for his friends, our Lord then called his disciples "friends" (Jn 15:13-15; cf. Lk 12:4). Thereby he revealed the heart of the God who spoke to Moses as to a friend (Ex 33:11) and to whom the patriarch Abraham was friend (2 Chron 20:7; Is 41:8; Jas 2:23).

In a less direct manner, we might connect the affection expressed in the word *storge* with the biblical God, in that the narrative repeatedly speaks about the divine compassion. At the centre of the faith of the Hebrew community stood a declaration of God's compassion, which the Book of Exodus describes as having its source in God himself. After revealing the divine name to Moses on Mount Sinai, Yahweh declares, "the compassionate and gracious God, slow to anger, abounding in love and faithfulness" (Ex 34:6; cf. Neh 9:17; Ps 111:4; 116:5; 86:15; 103:8; 145:8; Joel 2:13; Jon 4:2; Is 54:10). This God is compassionate in spite of human rebellion (Dan 9:9) and apart from our merit (Ex 33:19; Dan 9:18; Rom 9:15-16, 18).

Jesus appeals to God's ways to enjoin a similar compassion in the lives of his disciples: "You have heard that it was said, 'Love your neighbour and hate your enemy.' But I tell you: Love your enemies and pray for those who persecute you, that you may be sons of your Father in heaven. He causes his sun to rise on the evil and the good, and sends rain on the righteous and the unrighteous" (Mt 5:43-45; see also the parable of the good Samaritan, Lk 10:30-37). Our Lord's own life comprises a vivid illustration of this principle.

As Jesus' words suggest, in the biblical writings divine compassion draws from the familial imagery often connected with *storge*. This is evident in the story that is perhaps the most moving illustration of God's compassion, the parable of the prodigal son. While the wayward son "was still a long way off," Jesus declared, the father saw him "and was filled with compassion for him" (Lk 15:20). In a similar manner, Jeremiah describes God as desiring to have compassion on Ephraim, "my dear son" (Jer 31:20). And although the Old Testament narrative foundation for divine compassion may actually have been in the idea of God's covenant faithfulness, the original derivation of the Hebrew term "compassion" (*racham*) also carries the idea of family relations. Because the word's linguistic stem means "womb," compassion could be seen as referring to "the feeling of those born from the same womb" or "the love of a mother for her child."[38]

Meanings associated with *storge* and *philia* may claim a basis in the biblical narrative. But what about *eros*?[39] Here we step onto thinner ice. Christian thinkers readily admit the role of "desire" in not only human sexual relations, but even in religious devotion. In fact, there is a long-standing tradition that draws from the experience of longing and desire as forming the foundation for the quest for God. But is there any sense in which we can predicate *eros* of God?

We must admit up front that any attempt to do so is fraught with theological danger. Linking God with *eros* risks undermining the great truth that God is complete within the eternal community of the triune life and hence that creation is a non-necessary act. As a result, any *eros* within God cannot be in the form of a desire for creation borne from personal need.

Having said this, we must also acknowledge that one powerful motif in the biblical narrative of God's love for his people draws from marital love. The Old Testament prophets describe God's relationship to Israel through a three act drama. Act One consists of the betrothal of Israel to Yahweh. The loving God intended that Israel respond to his love like a virgin bride who gives herself willingly, continually and exclusively to her husband (Jer 2:2) and thereby becomes his delight (Is 62:5). Hence, rather than the typical ancient understanding which carried connotations of a contract between king and vassals, God's covenant with his people was to be a relationship of mutual love.

Act Two speaks about Israel's unfaithfulness. Yahweh's bride showed herself to be an adulterous spouse, forsaking her husband for other lovers. As a consequence, Yahweh "gave faithless Israel her certificate of divorce and sent her away because of all her adulteries" (Jer 3:8; cf. Hos 2:2, 4-5). Despite Israel's adultery, in the glorious third act the loving God proved his faithfulness.

The faithful love of Israel's husband formed the basis for the hope of a future restoration. Hence, through Hosea, God resolutely declares, "I will show my love to the one I called 'Not my loved one.' I will say to those called 'Not my people' 'You are my people'; and they will say, 'You are my God'" (Hos 2:23).

The New Testament writers such as Paul (Rom 9:25) and Peter (1 Pet 2:9-10) apply this dramatic motif of marital love to God's relationship with his new people. But they generally shift the imagery to speak more specifically about Christ and the church. Through his self-sacrificial life and death, Christ, the loving bridegroom (Mk 2:18-20; Jn 3:29; Rev 21:9), demonstrated his love for the church (Eph 5:32). In this manner the New Testament brought the marital drama into the broader, overarching narrative of the loving God who sends Jesus Christ to die for sinful humans.

The marital narrative raises a critical theological question: How can we affirm the erotic aspect of the divine love it embodies without falling into the trap of making God dependent on creation? Although we did not note it earlier, the same potential difficulty arises—even if less obviously—from our discussion of storge and philia. Our earlier treatment of the theological foundation for agape points toward the answer. Together with agape, we must lodge these concepts within, and bring them together in the divine Trinitarian life.

The love dynamic within the triune God is, of course, primarily *agape* [self-giving love], as John declares. Throughout eternity the Father gives his life to the Son. And as Jesus' obedience to his heavenly Father revealed, the Son eternally reciprocates that love in an eternal act of self-giving. In this manner, the divine essence is *agape*, an essence concretized in the Holy Spirit.

Yet the eternal love is infused with the other dimensions as well. This relationship includes the familial affection shared by Father and Son, as the Trinitarian language itself embodies. And we can readily understand that it involves the friendship enjoyed by eternal Friends as well.

But might we even venture to suggest that the inner-Trinitarian relationship also involves *eros*? To this query we answer "yes," provided we understand *eros* in its deeper sense of the desire for communion with the beloved.[40] Thus, Trinitarian *eros* is the reciprocal holy desire of the eternal Persons for communion with each other. Indeed, throughout his earthly life, Jesus demonstrated that he shares a unique communion with the one he called "Abba." The evangelists linked Christ's communion with his Father, in turn, with his glorification. This is evident, for example, in what is often called Jesus' "high priestly" prayer: "Father, I want those you have given me to be with me where I am, and to see my glory, the glory you have given me because you loved me before the creation of the world" (Jn 17:24). Here Jesus suggests that the intimacy of love the Father showers upon the Son—the communion they share—is the Son's glory. And it is precisely this glorious communion with the Father that we will eternally enjoy through the Son on the day of our eschatological glorification.[41]

Toward a Christian Theological Ethic of Love

These considerations suggest that while retaining the primacy of *agape* our conception of divine love must incorporate aspects of the other terms as well. Indeed, when stripped of the dimensions of love expressed in *philia* and *storge* our conception of the God who is *agape* can easily degenerate into a barren, distant, Stoic deity, who rescues humans for no other reason than because it is his "job" to do so. Repeatedly, theologians have been guilty of projecting a dispassionate God who is unmoved by his awareness of the human situation but is dutibound to save. The biblical God, in contrast, is *compassionate*. And this God *longs* to reconcile sinful humans who are at enmity with him, thereby transforming them into his friends, and to bring them into fellowship with himself as members of his eternal family (hence the tone of emotion in 2 Cor 5:20).

In the same way, our Christian ethic of love, with its focus on humans living out the divine image, ought to give place to all dimensions of the one concept of love, albeit as ruled and guided by *agape*. And all four aspects will be present in all relationships, yet in a form appropriate to each and always with *agape* at the centre. James Nelson states the rationale well: "If we define Christian love as agape or self-giving alone—without elements of desire, attraction, self-fulfillment, receiving—we are describing a love which is both impoverished and impoverishing. But the other elements of love without agape are ultimately self-destructive."[42]

An obvious example of the interaction of *agape* with the other three dimensions of love is that of human sexual relations within marriage. God's intention is clearly that *eros*, present in the form of sexual desire, play a central role in the joining together of man and woman to become "one flesh." Rather than deprecating the physical aspect of marital relations, as certain Christian thinkers have done, the biblical writers even celebrate the erotic dimension (e.g., Song of Songs; cf. 1 Cor 7:3-5; Heb 13:4). Yet the erotic cannot serve as the sole—or even the centre—foundation for a healthy marriage. The other aspects of love—friendship and affection—are equally important. But above all, the controlling dimension must be *agape* expressed through the mutual submission Paul cites as the foundation for his discussion of the ideal marriage (Eph 5:21). Whenever *eros* triumphs over *agape*, which is the case, for example, when unmarried couples engage in the sex act (e.g., adultery), unethical relationships emerge.[43]

A second example is that of care giving. The recent increased interest in this dynamic has netted a new model of ethics as "care."[44] Yet the idea is not new, for medical personnel have steadfastly defined themselves under the rubric of care.

In its care-giving function, medical ethicists have pinpointed the foundational principles of respect for patient autonomy and justice. In addition, health care professionals have traditionally committed themselves to cultivate the virtues of beneficence ("do good") and non-maleficence ("do no harm"). Beauchamp and Childress, for example, declare that although these principles "do not provide a complete system for general normative ethics, they do provide a sufficiently comprehensive framework for biomedical ethics."[45]

Medical personnel have repeatedly practised these virtues at great personal cost. Their self-sacrificial actions in the pursuit of their vocation have led many in our society to revere health care professionals as examples of the kind of self-giving love the biblical writers speak of through the use of the term *agape*. Medical professionals dare not lose this focus on an agapaic ethic. Indeed, *agape* ought to remain the controlling understanding of love within any ethic of care.

Yet the elevation of beneficence/non-maleficence as the central virtue of health care ethics and as the defining virtue of an agapaic ethic for caregivers risks allowing the patient-caregiver relationship to degenerate into an austere paternalism. Paternalism does not always take the form generally discussed by medical ethicists, namely, actions in which medical personnel override the principle of respect for the patient's autonomy. Also devastating to the professional-patient relationship is the paternalism in which health care professionals fulfil their duties in an aloof or condescending—and hence "uncaring"—manner.

Our use of "uncaring" in this context reminds us that in colloquial speech, the word "care" carries emotional overtones, as is also evidenced when we blurt out, "You don't care!" Such colloquial uses are not without consequence. They keep before us the widely-held conviction that true care giving includes an emotional component.

Contemporary ethicists acknowledge this whenever they appeal to the concept of compassion to provide the foundation for an ethic of care. The term itself means literally "to suffer with," which leads to the standard dictionary definition of compassion as "a sympathetic emotion created by the misfortunes of another accompanied by a desire to help."[46] Such compassion mirrors the compassionate God revealed in the biblical narrative, as well as the example of Jesus who willingly offered his healing touch to the medical outcasts of his day (Mk 1:41). As the evangelist points out, our Lord was not moved by a sense of duty, but by compassion. Consequently, care borne from a sympathetic heart is in accordance with the biblical call to us to reflect the divine character in our relationships with all people (Job 30:25; Col 3:12; Heb 13:3; 1 Pet 3:8) and thereby to act as true neighbours to those in need (Lk 10:25-37).

The presence of emotion—e.g., compassion—is crucial to the medical profession. In the context of a complete lack of emotional connection to the patient, even the best actions motivated by a concern to uphold beneficence and non-maleficence all too readily become mechanical, the professional caregiver becomes "merely a professional," and care giving becomes devoid of "care." To cite Paul's poetic words, "If I give all I possess to the poor and surrender my body to the flames, but have not love, I gain nothing" (1 Cor 13:3).

Compassionate care, however, may not always be triggered by a commitment to an agapaic ethic. *Agape*, the act of giving of oneself for the sake of the other, can all to readily be understood in a narrow, dutibound manner. Such "love" devoid of emotion may actually lead to the very paternalism that medical professionals need to avoid. As James Childress remarks negatively, "Paternalism clearly rests on the principle of love for the neighbor in our religious traditions and on the duty to benefit the patient in the Hippocratic tradition of medicine."[47]

As a solution to this problem, Childress calls for devising "practices and procedures that can indicate care and concern."[48] Stating the point more directly, the genesis of true professional care lies in a love that goes beyond giving of oneself for the sake of the other as motivated by a sense of duty. It involves an *agape* infused with a kind of affection for the patient that approaches what is found between family members (i.e., *storge*). Or put in Christian theological terms, the kind of love that lies at the heart of the Christian agapaic ethic is an *agape* informed by an affection for the other person, whom we view as a participant in the one human family and hence whom God created with the goal of participating in God's eternal community. As the Holy Spirit mixes such affection plus a sincere desire to enjoy the friendship of (*philia*) and true communion with (*eros*) the other person in God's eternal fellowship with the self-giving impulse (*agape*), the Spirit of the relation between the Father and the Son leads us into the fullness of the Christian love ethic. It is this kind of comprehensive love that characterizes the truly *Christian* caregiver.

◆ ◆ ◆ ◆

Don and Donna took action. Over dinner one evening they discussed the situation openly, concluding that they had been confusing their desire for friendship and true communion borne out of a growing affection for each other with sexual desire. While not wanting to eliminate all physical expressions, they committed themselves to enjoy the deeper aspects of their relationship uncluttered by the guilt that engaging in sexual intercourse might introduce, abstaining, that is, until such a time as they had committed themselves to each other in a lifelong partnership.

◆ ◆ ◆ ◆

George's family physician dropped by to see him today. From their brief conversation, Dr. Hodge sensed the anxiety in the voice of his patient of many years. Carefully and slowly, the doctor explained to George the prognosis for his future and the steps the two of them would take together to insure a full recovery. Abruptly, George asked Dr. Hodge about his golf game.

Notes

1 All scriptural quotations in this article are taken from the New International version of the Bible, copyright the New York International Bible Society.

2 M. A. Reid, "Theological Virtues," in *New Dictionary of Christian Ethics and Pastoral Theology*, ed. David J. Atkinson et al. (Downers Grove, Ill.: InterVarsity, 1995), 844.

3 For a helpful discussion of the double command, see Rudolf Schnackenburg, *The Moral Teaching of the New Testament*, trans. J. Holland-Smith and W. J. O'Hara (New York: Seabury, 1965), 90–109.

4 Schnackenburg, *Moral Teaching of the New Testament*, 106.

5 So claims Wolfgang Schrage, *The Ethics of the New Testament*, trans. David E. Green (Philadelphia: Fortress, 1988), 70.

6 C. S. Lewis, *The Four Loves*, (London: Collins, Fontana Books edition, 1963). William Barclay [*New Testament Words* (London: S. C. M., 1964), 17–18] is in fundamental agreement with Lewis. However, Paul Tillich's love quadrilateral begins with *epithumia* (desire) rather than *storge* [*Love, Power and Justice: Ontological Analysis and Ethical Applications*, Galaxie Books edition (New York: Oxford, 1960), 28]. This may suggest that no one list is exhaustive.

7 The adjective *philostorgos* does occur once (Rom 12:10). See Barclay, *New Testament Words*, 18.

8 Ibid.

9 Gustav Staehlin, "Phileo," in *Theological Dictionary of the New Testament*, ed. Gerhard Friedrich, trans. Geoffrey W. Bromiley (Grand Rapids, Mich.: Eerdmans, 1974), 9:136.

10 Staehlin, "*phileo*," TDNT, 9:116.

11 Ibid., 128, 134.

12 Perhaps the most significant statement is Anders Nygren, *Agape and Eros*, trans. Philip S. Watson (Philadelphia: Westminster, 1953).

13 Ethelbert Stauffer, "*agapao*," TDNT, 1:35.

14 Ibid., 35–36.

15 See, for example, Paul Ramsey, *Basic Christian Ethics* (New York: Charles Scribner's Sons, 1950). For a short discussion of why Christian language chose *agape* over the other terms, see Barclay, *New Testament Words*, 20–21.

16 Stauffer writes, "The examples of *agape* thus far adduced are few in number, and in many cases doubtful or hard to date. "*agapao*," TDNT, 1:37.

17 Barclay, *New Testament Words*, 20.

18 Ibid., 21.

19 Stauffer, "*agapao*," TDNT, 1:36–37.

20 Schrage, *Ethics of the NT*, 206–7.

21 J. Paul Sampley, *Walking Between the Times: Paul's Moral Reasoning* (Minneapolis, Minn.: Fortress, 1991), 37–43.

22 John Knox concludes that for Paul, love "belongs essentially within the Christian community and has meaning there which it cannot have outside." *The Ethic of Jesus in the Teaching of the Church* (Nashville, Tenn.: Abingdon, 1961), 92.

23 Victor Paul Furnish, *Theology and Ethics in Paul* (Nashville, Tenn.: Abingdon, 1968), 233.

24 See, for example, Jack T. Sanders, *Ethics in the New Testament: Change and Development* (Philadelphia: Fortress, 1974), 56.

25 Ibid., 63.

26 Athanasius wrote, "Since the Father has given all things to the Son, he possesses all things afresh in the Son." *Apologia Contra Arian* 3.36, in *A Select Library of Nicene and Post-Nicene Fathers of the Christian Church*, vol. 4: *St. Athanasius: Select Works and Letters*, trans. Atkinson, ed. Archibald Robertson, 2nd ser. (Grand Rapids, Mich.: Eerdmans, 1975), 119.

27 Athanasius, *Contra Arian* 3.6, in *The Early Christian Fathers*, ed. and trans. Henry Bettenson, Oxford paperback edition (London: Oxford, 1969), 287.

28 Augustine, *The Trinity* 6.5.7, trans. Steven McKenna, vol. 45 of *The Fathers of the Church*, ed. Hermigild Dressler (Washington, D.C.: Catholic University of America Press, 1963), 206–7; see also 15.17.27; 5.11.12; 15.19.37. For the connection of this Augustinian idea to the Greek tradition, see Yves Congar, *I Be-*

lieve in the Holy Spirit, trans. David Smith, 3 vol. (New York: Seabury, 1983), 3:88–89, 147–48. For a contemporary delineation of this position, see David Coffey, "The Holy Spirit as the Mutual Love of the Father and the Son," *Theological Studies* 51 (1990): 193–229.

29 Augustine, *The Trinity* 15.17.27–29, 31 [491–94, 495–96]; 15.19.37 [503–504].

30 Lewis, *Four Loves*, 117.

31 Tillich, *Love, Power, and Justice*, 116.

32 Lewis, *Four Loves*, 125.

33 Ibid., 122.

34 Tillich's critique of the "lower" forms of love moved from the acknowledgement that they in fact are "different qualities of the one nature of love" which he sees as an ontological category. *Love, Power, and Justice*, 24–28.

35 See, for example, James B. Nelson, *Embodiment* (Minneapolis, Minn.: Augsburg, 1978), 110–14; James B. Nelson, *Body Theology* (Louisville, Ky.: Westminster/John Knox, 1992), 22.

36 Tillich, *Love, Power, and Justice*, 118–19.

37 Gilbert C. Meilaender, *Friendship: A Study in Theological Ethics* (Notre Dame, Ind.: University of Notre Dame Press, 1981), 18.

38 Elizabeth R. Achtemeier, "Mercy, Merciful; Compassion; Pity," in the *Interpreter's Dictionary of the Bible*, ed. George Arthur Buttrick (New York: Abingdon, 1962), 3:352.

39 Nelson is among those contemporary voices who are offering an unconditional affirmative response to this question: "Of particular importance in our time is the reclaiming of the much-neglected, much-feared *erotic* dimensions of love." *Body Theology*, 23.

40 For a discussion of *eros* as communion, see Nelson, *Embodiment*, 34–35, 110, 112.

41 For a short discussion of this, see Stanley J. Grenz, *Theology for the Community of God* (Nashville, Tenn.: Broadman & Holman, 1994), 844–45.

42 Nelson, *Embodiment*, 113.

43 For a fuller delineation of this point, see Stanley J. Grenz, *Sexual Ethics* (Dallas: Word, 1990), 81–98.

44 See, for example, Nel Noddlings, *Care: A Feminine Approach to Ethics and Moral Education* (Berkeley: University of California Press, 1984).

45 Tom L. Beauchamp and James F. Childress, *Principles of Biomedical Ethics* (New York: Oxford, 1989), 15.

46 *New Webster's Dictionary of the English Language*, rev. ed. (1981), s.v. "Compassion."

47 James F. Childress, *Priorities in Biomedical Ethics* (Philadelphia: Westminster, 1981), 23.

48 Childress, *Priorities in Biomedical Ethics*, 32–33.

Arnold Voth

Physician Beneficence, Patient Autonomy, and Christian Values

In preparation for this paper, I researched about fifteen years of back issues of both the Canadian and the US CMDS publications looking for material. Though the subjects of autonomy and beneficence are indeed mentioned from time to time in other discussions, they have never been discussed directly. This is surprising, in view of the fact that both of them probably lie at the heart of our society's debates over the related issues of abortion and euthanasia. I am greatly honoured to be asked to present the premier discourse on autonomy and beneficence during this conference.

Questions for Reflection
1. Is the physician's primary responsibility always to do good?
2. Should the mentally competent patient always have the last word on his treatment?
3. Is there sometimes a conflict between the above two goals?

Case Histories
Case #1

Mr. R., a thirty-two-year-old male, HIV-positive, presents to the emergency room with acute pneumonia that turns out to be Pneumocystis carinii, a common complication of AIDS. Mr. R. produces a living will designating a durable health care proxy and specifically forbidding cardiopulmonary resuscitation or endotracheal intubation under any circumstances. His physician, Dr. D., assures him that his wishes will be respected. Dr. D. orders the appropriate antibiotics, leaves the room, and returns again just in time to see his patient in acute respiratory distress with a bright red rash, clearly an anaphylactic reaction to the antibiotic. This complication can almost certainly be successfully treated within hours. But if the patient is to survive, he *must* be intubated at once to restore the patency of his airways while it is still possible to pass a tube through the rapidly swelling tissues of mouth and pharynx. The living will specifically prohibits such intervention. What should Dr. D. do?[1]

Case #2
Mrs. M., an otherwise healthy thirty-four-year-old woman presents to the emergency room with increasingly severe abdominal pain suggestive of an acute appendicitis. She is perfectly rational, mentally competent, and logical; however, she has an irrational fear of surgery and flatly refuses any suggestion of an operation, believing that she'll never wake up! Every effort is made by physicians, nurses, and other personnel to understand her phobia and talk her out of it, but to no avail. She remains adamantly opposed to surgery. At first, efforts are made to accommodate her wishes and she is treated with high-dose antibiotics in the hope that the appendicitis will settle with conservative treatment alone. But she continues to deteriorate, and soon becomes delirious with the mounting fever and septicemia. All of her family are out of town and cannot be reached until the next day at the earliest. Should her physicians operate despite her explicit refusal of surgery? Or should they respect her wishes, only to let her die of septicemia?[2]

These two cases are not everyday medicine, but they do illustrate that the twin concepts of physician beneficence and patient autonomy are not always matched horses that trot together in perfect rhythm. They may be a couple of stallions galloping in opposite directions.

Definitions

Although the principles of beneficence, nonmaleficence, autonomy, and distributive justice have been recognized as the four cardinal virtues of medical ethics for most of this century, this has not always been the case. The oldest of these virtues is physician beneficence, for it was at the heart of Hippocratic medicine. Physician beneficence means simply that the physician will always do what is good for the patient, her life and her health. All diagnostic interventions, treatment, and information provided are chosen to maximize the patient's medical benefits. This, rather than pleasing the patient, is the physician's primary goal. On the other hand, however, this does not mean that the patient may not participate in decision-making, or that his consent will not be sought. What it does mean is that when there is a conflict between the patient's wishes and what the practitioner assumes to be the best possible medical treatment, the physician prevails. Indeed, in Hippocratic medicine, the physician had the right and the duty to present information in a way that encouraged the patient to choose the best course of action. If need be, the physician would withhold information or even deceive the patient to achieve the best possible outcome.

Autonomy is a term derived from the Greek *autos* meaning *self*, and *nomos* meaning *rule, governance,* or *law*.

Patient autonomy is a much more recent concept than physician beneficence—in fact, it was a concept unknown to Hippocrates and his colleagues. This principle states that the mentally competent patient will always have the last word on her health care. She is free to seek care as she desires, receive as much or as little help as she desires, or ignore her physician's advice altogether. The physician is obligated to yield to the patient's wishes, regardless of whether he believes them to be wise or foolish.

Christian values do not necessarily mirror any or all of the cardinal virtues of medical ethics, but they do share many common principles that I will outline later in this lecture.

A History of the Concepts of Beneficence and Autonomy

Hippocratic medicine was built on the concept of physician beneficence. In his book, *The New Medicine: Life and Death after Hippocrates* Nigel Cameron states:

> Firstly, we note that some kind of ethical "paternalism" is fundamental to the Hippocratic concept of medicine. The Hippocratic physician engages to practise a specific kind of medicine; not whatever kind of medicine the marketplace demands. His interest is not primarily in how his patient sees things; and he finds it impossible

to believe that his patient's true interests could actually lie in any other direction than that to which by oath he is committed.[3]

Beauchamp, in another article on beneficence in the Hippocratic model comments:

> The Corpus Hippocraticum fails to address today's problems of the autonomy of patients. Rather, it bluntly advises physicians of the wisdom of "concealing most things from the patient, while you are attending to him . . . turning his attention away from what is being done to him; . . . revealing nothing of the patient's future or present condition." In these writings the physician is generally portrayed as one who commands and decides, while patients are conceived as persons who must place themselves in the physician's hands and obey commands . . . The purpose of medicine expressed in this tradition is that of benefiting the sick and keeping them from harm and injustice.[4]

The beneficence model of medical ethics held almost unchallenged sway until modern times, in both writings on ethics and in codes of ethics for physicians worldwide. In the 1960s, various civil rights movements changed the face of bioethics. When applied to the practice of medicine the idea of a rights-based ethic clashed with the Hippocratic model of beneficence. The dawn of the patient autonomy movement changed the paradigm of ethics from a physician-based model of beneficence to a patient-based model of autonomy. At first, medicine sailed through the transition in the sublime belief that autonomy was just another parameter being added to the practice of medicine. Not until the conflicts over abortion and euthanasia did we realize that these two principles are sometimes at odds with each other.

If you give priority to the beneficent model of medical ethics, you will have no problem with either of the two case histories I have cited. You will simply act in what you believe to be the obvious best interests of the patient. Similarly, if you give precedence to the autonomy model of ethics, you will have no problem. You will simply follow the dictates of the patient, accepting his demise as the direct consequence of his decision, rather than because of any failure on your part. But if you regard both principles as equally important, you have a problem. And that problem is at the core of this paper.

Current View of Beneficence and Autonomy

The beneficence model of medical ethics views all of the physician's actions in the light of their benefit to the patient's well-being. From the moment of the first encounter with the patient, the physician's goal is to determine what may benefit the patient's health the most effectively. The autonomy model, on the other hand, views all of the physician's actions in the light of their relation to the patient's desires. The interview and subsequent interventions are thus aimed at discovering what it is the patient wishes to know and to have done.

Today, the autonomy model prevails in all contemporary ethical teaching; the physician is seen as beneficent when she fulfils the patient's wishes. Thomas Murray has said rather aptly that "Autonomy sometimes appears to be regarded as a kind of universal moral solvent."[5] When I presented the two case histories I used at the beginning of this lecture to a random sampling of friends and asked them for their advice, almost all of them began by saying something like, "Of course, you *must* respect the patient's wishes!" They then proceeded to consider how to get patients to change their minds. Hippocrates would have enjoyed listening to them! None of them even considered the alternative of simply ignoring the patient's wishes. They felt, as you probably did, that autonomy was like the Ten Commandments that admitted no change. But at the same time, they also felt uncomfortable with the end result of this view. The students and residents whom I teach daily are almost incapable of thinking in the "beneficent" mode of ethics, and therefore find themselves trapped in a major bioethical "Catch-22."

In real clinical life, the apparent conflict between the two models is not as absolute as I have indicated. Every physician tries to be as beneficent as possible, even while she seeks the patient's decision on treatment alternatives. Beneficence does not rule out a large measure of patient autonomy in modern clinical practice. Patients do not expect absolute autonomy either. They certainly expect to have the last word on whether major treatment plans or surgery are undertaken. However, when a patient presents to the emergency room in a state of hysterical agitation, no one would argue that the choice of initial sedative therapy is best left to the physician. Modern clinical practice blends physician beneficence, often described as paternalistic, with patient autonomy.

There are, however, two good reasons for separating these principles in our discussion today. First, it is much easier to clothe our feelings and convictions in understandable terms when we deal with one concept at a time. Second, we must separate them in order to analyze their past contributions to ethical thinking and to try to predict their future effects on ethical thinking and decision-making. Since we are all a part of the ethical trends of our day, it is our duty to try to foresee what the long-term result of following this or the other practice may be. To do this, we must dissect the twin virtues of beneficence and autonomy as though they were separate and unrelated.

Autonomy: Is It Really the Ultimate Moral Value?

For many people today, autonomy is not only the most important of the cardinal virtues of medical ethics; it is the *only* virtue. Popular thinking is that if only the patient is allowed to choose freely among available alternatives, is given whatever he wants, and is not asked to do what he does not want to do; all will be well. Because autonomy is the rallying cry of the proponents of abortion on demand and euthanasia, it merits our most careful study.

The Autonomous Decision

For an autonomous decision to be made, several conditions must be met. First, the individual making the decision must be an autonomous individual: that is, somebody with enough mental competence to assess the situation, and able to carry out that decision or make someone else to carry it out for them. A slave, for example, may well be a competent decision-maker; but because he lacks the power to carry out his decision, he is not autonomous. Second, the individual must possess sufficient information to make a rational decision. Third, she must be able to process this information adequately. This processing involves more complex matters than just knowing the facts, especially considering that one's health or life is at stake. We do not make our decisions in a vacuum: we make them in the context of a community. When told she has a malignancy, a patient rarely makes a swift and completely independent treatment decision. She will first share the diagnosis with her family, her family physician, close friends, and so on, and then begin to process the meaning of possible treatment alternatives as she continues to interact with her community. The final decision is autonomous, but the process of arriving at it requires this community. In the absence of such community, autonomy becomes difficult because the individual has trouble processing the information in isolation from his community.

Looking back at our case histories in the light of these points, we realize why the two patients had problems arriving at satisfactory autonomous decisions. The HIV-positive man did not know that he might develop a highly treatable and reversible complication of treatment for which artificial respiration would be a very effective and very short term necessity. As a result, his decision, although certainly autonomous, didn't include this possibility. The woman with appendicitis, like Mr. R., was mentally competent but unlike him, was well-informed. Unfortunately, she lacked the community which could have helped her process this information. She also had an irrational fear that prevented her from making a reasonable decision. Irrational phobias make rational decisions impossible. In a very limited sense, then, she was not mentally competent, although globally she certainly was competent.

There is a certain inherent, simple justice about self-determination and autonomy that appeals to us naturally and easily. Autonomy remains the most vital moral bulwark against oppression of all kinds. In the *Hastings Report*, Thomas Murray asserts that, "Wherever the powerful seek to impose their will on the powerless, autonomy, along with justice, should be our battle cry."[6] But the concept of autonomy has its limits, and we should explore them carefully before we too are lead unwittingly to accept it as a "universal moral solvent."

The Limits of the Autonomous Decision
What then might be the limits and weaknesses of a society that accepts the autonomous decision as the ultimate moral good?

First, a truly autonomous decision takes no account either of the needs of others, nor of the individual's need for others. It is based

206 • Arnold Voth

solely on the needs and wants of the individual making the decision. The principle of autonomy teaches us nothing about living with others, even though community forms the largest part of our lives. From the time of birth until death the individual is situated in a family, as well as in other types of communities: workplace, residential, religious, academic, and so on. Our life has very little meaning without such grounding in community. Why then, would we want to make decisions in complete isolation from such communities? Is not truly autonomous decision-making somewhat analogous to planning a garden without considering the available soil or the weather or the surrounding vegetation or the wants of those who may wish to benefit from the garden?

Second, an autonomous decision takes no account of the autonomy of those individuals whose help may be needed to achieve that decision. For example, the patient who demands the right to an assisted suicide does not take into account the moral autonomy of the individual charged with assisting the action. A woman claiming the right to an abortion under any circumstances takes no account of the autonomy of the health care personnel whose assistance will have to be coerced to achieve her desire.

Third, the concept of total autonomy takes no account of the realities of life. There is no such thing as totally autonomous decision-making. Most of the decisions I must make impinge on someone else's life in some way. If I value that other person, I must involve her in making my decisions. Furthermore, much of my decision-making must take into account what is possible for me and society. I cannot have everything, and society is under no obligation to give me everything. In this sense, the concept of true autonomy ends up being a false prophet: it promises what it can never deliver. In real life, of course, most of us are rational enough to consider our communities in our decision-making. We involve our family, we involve our caregivers, we involve our neighbours when appropriate, we consider what society may reasonably be asked to give us. This process clearly does not permit autonomous decision-making. Why, then, should we place so much value on an ethical principle which we will mostly ignore in real life?

Fourth, the concept of total autonomy depends heavily on the goodwill, integrity, and trust of the physician, but without actually acknowledging it. If you are my patient, you depend on me to listen carefully to your problem, to put my heart and mind enthusiastically to the solution for your problem, to obtain from the health care system what you need to remedy your problem, and to explain all of this to you so that you can make an intelligent decision. The principle of autonomy, however, takes no account of this complex interaction between physician and patient. It simply assumes that whatever you want, you will get because it's your decision. This attitude is an insidious problem because it is completely out of step with reality. Particularly in my area of internal medicine, how much I am able to do for a patient depends on the enthusiasm, creativity, and zest that I can find in myself to hear, examine, and solve his problem. In an atmosphere of mutual trust and confidence these qualities come forth naturally and easily enough. But every physician knows that the surest way a patient can shut off the flow of these qualities in the practitioner is for her to arrive in the consulting room flanked by a glaring spouse, an angry in-law, and a defiant daughter for a collective delivery of a "these are my rights and you had better deliver them" speech. This vigorous assertion of autonomy promptly dries up the physician's fount of enthusiasm and, instead, shifts her focus to defending what has been done and defining what must be done. In real life, what I am obligated to do is far less effective than what I could do if I applied my heart and mind enthusiastically to the task. Thus the concept of total autonomy taken to its logical conclusion ends up sabotaging the medical care of the autonomous individual. It teaches a patient nothing about developing a fruitful physician-patient relationship. What it does teach tends to destroy such a relationship rather than to build it. Once again, autonomy ends up being a false prophet by promising what it cannot possibly deliver: the best possible medical care that a physician is capable of providing.

Fifth, the concept of complete autonomy takes no account of the realities of clinical practice. Fully autonomous decision-making by patients would quickly reduce the efficiency of the average hospital to the stalling point. It is simply unrealistic to believe that the patient can be involved in potentially every aspect of decision-making about his care in a busy hospital. There will never be the time to review with the patient the dozens of decisions that must be made every day with respect to his treatment. Patient autonomy is therefore not the "universal moral solvent" that eliminates all ethical problems, nor is it the ultimate moral imperative.

Beneficence: The Ultimate Moral Imperative?

The Beneficence Model of Medical Ethics

The autonomy model of medical ethics states simply that the patient's wishes must be given precedence over all other considerations when there is a conflict between patient and caregiver. The beneficence model, on the other hand, states that the well-being of the patient takes precedence over all other considerations. Under the autonomy model, both of our patients in the case histories would have been allowed to die for lack of the treatment which they refused. In contrast, under the beneficence model, both would have been treated on the grounds that their physical well-being would have been best served by the physician's decision and not their own.

The Benefits of Beneficence

In view of our case histories, therefore, the advantages of the beneficence model are worth careful study.

First, it represents the core of belief and teaching on medical ethics. The practice of medicine is built on the idea of beneficence rather than patient autonomy. A few years ago, Dickstein and others studied 141 pledges received from all US medical schools accredited in 1989.[7] Very few of these oaths mentioned respect for patient autonomy. None of them pledged the physician to tell the truth to his patient at all times, whereas over half of them mentioned beneficence and nonmaleficence. Physicians are familiar with and have been dedicated to the principle of beneficence for over two thousand years. It is the principle they understand best.

Second, the principle of beneficence places the ultimate responsibility for decision-making in the hands of the individual best informed about the matter at hand. Do not dismiss this as overweening paternalism. We all live with such "beneficence" models very happily elsewhere in life. During a recent vacation to the tiny Himalayan mountain kingdom of Bhutan, we approached the airport at Paro during a vicious windstorm. As our aircraft pitched, tossed, rolled, and plunged repeatedly into air pockets with heart-stopping suddenness, the pilot never once asked our opinions about whether he should proceed with a landing or risk running out of fuel looking for an alternate airport. I'm very glad that he didn't, for even with the best explanations, none of us would have been qualified to offer him reasonable advice. We simply trusted the pilot. Happily, he justified our trust by executing an absolutely flawless landing right into the teeth of the windstorm. He received a thunderous ovation from the cabin for his efforts! If we unhesitatingly accept decision-making on our behalf by those most qualified to do it elsewhere, why shouldn't we accept it in medicine?

Third, the beneficence model simplifies decision-making for the physician. The purpose of medicine in this model is to benefit the sick, to restore them to health as well as possible, and to keep them from harm and injustice either at their own hands or at the hands of others who may wish to injure them. The model certainly allows for decision-making by the patient, but when the patient's decision, in his doctor's opinion, is not in his own best interests, it grants him the right to overrule the patient's conclusion. It focuses the physician's mind on how best to solve a problem of restoring health, rather than on pleasing the patient.

Fourth, the beneficence model encourages the highest standards of integrity and care by the physician. The caregiver who realizes that the patient's well-being is always the goal of all diagnostics and treatment has a much higher sense of purpose than the physician who is made to feel like a waitress taking orders. One who merely takes orders in turn takes no responsibility for the health of her clients. After all, every oath of professional responsibility is based on the beneficence model of ethics. What is the point of "always doing good" if the final decision for good or bad rests with the patient?

The Possible Maleficence of Beneficence

The beneficence model, however, has its problems as well. First, it has fallen on hard times in the twentieth century. It would be difficult, if not impossible, to follow it completely in our society. Self-determination is such an important part of our Western way of thinking that the old style of paternalistic medicine simply will not work. People regard decisions about their health much differently than they do the decisions of their pilot, their accountant, or their gardener. Health care professionals are certainly expected to be beneficent in the practice of their professions, but only as long as their decisions fall in line with the patient's wishes. When there is a conflict, beneficence is quickly dismissed as arrogant paternalism.

Second, the beneficence model is obviously open to endless abuse by the unscrupulous. True, the medical profession is committed to preventing such abuse by the nature of its commitment to the welfare of its patients, but that is only one check that has failed in the past. The evils of German medicine in the years leading up to the Nazi regime were initially justified on the principle of beneficence. Long before Hitler came to power, the involuntary euthanasia of the unfit was accepted by many compliant physicians who felt that such people would not want to live anyway. Had the principle of patient autonomy existed at that time, many of the worst abuses of medicine in Nazi Germany might have been avoided. The need to explain and justify treatment to the patient is a valuable check on the power of the medical profession, a stopgap that cannot possibly exist under a purely beneficent model of medical ethics.

Third, the principle of beneficence discourages the patient's accepting responsibility for his own health. In this sense the pilot-passenger relationship is very different from the doctor-patient relationship. The passenger cannot contribute anything useful to a safe landing, except perhaps his silence during the crisis! The patient, on the other hand, is capable of influencing his own health in a great many ways. His participation in his care, then, can only enhance his sense of responsibility for self.

Fourth, the beneficence model assumes that the caregiver actually knows what is best for the patient. One hopes that most of the time this will be true. In the cases cited at the beginning of this paper, for example, the best treatment options are obvious; this model poses no problem in these instances. But even the most arrogant physician will admit that there are many times when he does not know what is best for the patient. When a patient with cancer has the option of a few additional months of life at the cost of much suffering from aggressive therapy, do physicians know what is best for the patient in the context of her life and community? I doubt it.

Beneficence and Autonomy: A Summing Up

The twenty authors I reviewed on the subject of beneficence and autonomy in preparation for this lecture all seemed to agree on one thing: that neither model alone truly works within the framework of today's ethical environment. The autonomy model leaves no room for the needs of community life and sometimes exposes patients, such as those in our case histories, to grave dangers to their health because of the unforeseen or because of personal idiosyncrasies. The beneficence model, on the other hand, offers too little protection for the patient's desire for self-determination. What is needed is some sort of marriage of the two concepts so that one or the other may be given priority, depending on the situation. Just how this marriage is to be arranged is unclear in the writings I consulted. When should the physician set aside the patient's wishes and simply act in what he believes is his best interests? When should she set aside her wish to do the best thing for the patient's health and listen to his preference instead?

Autonomy, Beneficence, and Christian Values

What then, do Christian physicians and health professionals have to contribute to the issue of beneficence versus autonomy in patient care? I think we have a great deal to contribute, far more than most secular ethicists would guess. Not only do Christian values affirm what contemporary ethicists regard as almost sacred in respect to the twin virtues of beneficence and autonomy, but they also answer most of the fears arising from the unfettered use of these models.

Autonomy and Christian Values

The language of Christ and the New Testament as written by the Apostle Paul and his fellow writers reflects respect for individual autonomy. Christ invites all to come to him. He invites his disciples to follow him. He invites the sick, the weak, the hungry to experience his brand of healing. Christ does not use the language of coercion or compulsion anywhere in the Gospels; instead, he speaks of drawing all people to him. The best example of Christ's approach to the individual's autonomy occurs in the account of the healing at the Pool of Bethesda. Christ sees the paralytic and has pity on him, yet the paralytic does not ask him for healing as did the many who crowded around Jesus day after day. So Christ asks him gently, "Do you want to get well?" (Jn 5:1-9).[8]

In the secular world, respect for individual autonomy is encouraged because it is the current ethical fashion. For Christians, such respect is due because all people are created in the image of God. It is part of our sacred duty toward all of humankind. It arises out of the Christian belief in every individual's infinite worth before God.

The Abuse of Autonomy and Christian Values

Many secular writers worry that an exclusive emphasis on autonomy will lead to a collection of totally selfish individuals unable to live together in harmony. Thomas Murray writes:

> A near-exclusive emphasis on autonomy is attractive in part because it permits us to avoid many unpleasant and complex realities—the strains of living in communities in which others not only have different interests, but may be ornery and unreasonable besides; the gnawing difficulties and deep satisfactions of enduring family relationships; the confusing, embarrassing, and sometimes ugly particulars of the human psyche.[9]

Despite the New Testament's emphasis on respecting individual autonomy, it contains an equal emphasis on voluntarily giving up autonomy for others' sake. In the well-known discourses on eating meat offered to idols in Romans 14 and again in 1 Corinthians 8, the Apostle Paul sums up our duties toward one another: "Each of us should please his neighbour for his good, to build him up" (Rom 15:2). In a community where each individual is ever ready to surrender his autonomy for the sake of his brother or sister, abuse of autonomy becomes well-nigh impossible. Are we ready to demonstrate to our medical communities this kind of voluntary laying down of our autonomy for the sake of Christ and others? As patients? As physicians? As caregiver?

Beneficence and Christian Values

That beneficence is a Christian value scarcely needs to be repeated. It is also at the core of the Good News of Christ. Christ's life was a life of beneficence. We have been called to follow him in every respect, but especially in doing good for others. The foundation of Christian beneficence, however, is quite different from that of the Hippocratic beneficence. The latter is based on the assumption that the physician knows what is best for the patient and has a duty to do it, while Christian beneficence is based on our love for our fellow human beings. Both Christ and the Apostle Paul state in almost the same words: "'Love your neighbour as yourself.' Love does no harm to its neighbour. Therefore love is the fulfilment of the law" (Rom 13:9b, 10). Beneficence that arises out of love for the individual is much less likely to result in the caregiver's abuse of the trust that the patient places in him.

During a trek in the Himalayas in the tiny state of Sikkim two years ago, my friend Ron and I encountered another trekker from the south of India who was seriously ill with acute mountain sickness. He was travelling alone with a few porters and a guide. Dependent on the counsel of passers-by like us, since his judgment was considerably impaired and his demands often unreasonable, his rescue took several days longer than it should have taken. When we learned of this unfortunate man's near death due to the rescue effort's inept handling, Ron and I agreed that we would not like to do such a trek without the company of at least one friend. If things went wrong, only a friend would have the judgment to know when to ignore our requests, make decisions for us, and have the persistence to follow through with necessary rescue actions. Indeed, this is the kind of beneficence that the Christian is pledged to bring to anyone who approaches him in need.

Christian beneficence, however, should not only be practised out of one's sense of love for a friend: it should be practised out of one's obedience to God. We do for others whatever we would have them do for us, and we do this out of our obedience to Christ's commands to us. So while secular beneficence is based on the principle of professional noblesse oblige, Christian beneficence is based on deference to Christ and his Lordship.

Christian Values, Autonomy, and Community

One of the abiding fears of secular ethicists regarding the doctrine of autonomy is that an unbalanced acceptance of autonomy will destroy community. Murray expresses it thus:

> Because it touched such deep currents in American character and culture, autonomy cast a dazzling glow that many hoped would be able to illuminate all of the

dark corners of our shared moral life. Some still retain that faith; others, such as myself, believe that autonomy remains a vital moral bulwark against oppression, but that it is not an all-encompassing guide to living good lives or building good communities . . . communities that value love and loyalty and forgiveness as much as they value autonomy.[10]

The Christian church has a two-thousand year history of building community. You cannot read more than a few pages at a time anywhere in the New Testament without encountering some comment on the Christian duty to live together peaceably and harmoniously. Yet, it is always a duty that must be freely given out of love for our neighbour. This may be the best time of all for Christians in the health professions to model, for the secular world, a community life that still respects the autonomy of the individual.

Conclusion

Daniel Callahan, the long-standing President of the Hastings Centre for Bioethics notes that:

> Bioethics has displayed two serious deficiencies, exactly the kind that usually afflict golden children; it has failed to pursue with sufficient imagination the idea of the common good, or public interest, on the one hand, and that of personal responsibility, or the moral uses of individual choice, on the other. By its tendency to reduce the problem of the common good to justice, and the individual moral life to the gaining of autonomy, it has left a moral void.[11]

Secular bioethics has indeed left a moral void, but this is a space that Christ's teachings are more than sufficient to fill. It is up to us to model these teachings to frightened ethicists as well as to the world in general.

In my view, the Christian physician should not have much trouble with the two case histories presented at the beginning of this lecture. The young man with HIV could not have foreseen that he might develop a complication for which the short-term use of intubation and respiratory support would be most effective, with little risk of subsequently diminished function. A loving friend could easily make such a decision for him, and the Christian physician ought to be that loving friend. The woman with appendicitis was paralysed by an irrational fear. When our friends are paralysed by irrational fears, we take them by the hand and walk with them through their anxieties, even blindfolding them if we must. That is what this patient needed, and a Christian physician could have provided the care that she could not bring herself to accept. In the end, she was, in fact, taken to the operating room without her consent, survived easily, and never again mentioned her objection to surgery.

The uncritical acceptance of either the autonomy model or the beneficence model of medical ethics is fraught with many perils, and ethicists are justified in pointing them out to us. The Christian community has the opportunity to show the world how these conflicting models can be harnessed together for the good of the patient under the Lordship of our Saviour. God grant us the vision and the spiritual energy to seize this opportunity.

Notes

[1] L. M. Silverman and M. Dennis, "Whether No Means No," Commentary, *Hastings Centre Report* (May/June 1992): 26-27.

[2] A modification of a case history from personal communication.

[3] Nigel M. de S. Cameron, *The New Medicine: Life and Death after Hippocrates*, (Wheaton, Ill.: Crossway, 1991), 28.

[4] T. L. Beauchamp, "The Promise of the Beneficence Model for Medical Ethics," *Journal of Contemporary Health, Law & Policy* 6 (1990): 145-55.

[5] T. H. Murray, "Individualism and Community: The Contested Terrain of Autonomy," *Hastings Centre Report* 24 (1994): 32-33.

[6] Ibid., 32-33.

[7] E. Dickstein et al., "Ethical Principles Contained in Currently Professed Medical Oaths," *Academic Medicine* 66 (1991): 622-24.

[8] All scriptural quotations in this article are taken from the New International version of the Bible, copyright the New York International Bible Society.

[9] Murray, "Individualism and Community," 32-33.

[10] Ibid., 32-33.

[11] D. Callahan, "Bioethics: Private Choice and Common Good," *Hastings Centre Report* 24 (1994): 28-31.

Margaret M. Cottle

Care, a Basis for the Physician-Patient Relationship: "Who Is My Brother?"

"Care, a basis for the physician-patient relationship: 'Who is my brother?'" This is a challenging subject because of the variety of ideas as to precisely what constitutes caring for a patient. The concept of care will be examined from several perspectives. Principle-based and relational-based ethical systems will be discussed. An attempt will be made to articulate a biblical concept of caring, its foundations and distinctives, and its implications for Christian physicians and health care workers. How does or should our faith affect how we care for patients?

It would be best to begin with a disclaimer: I am completely out of my depth in this project. My understanding of bioethics is rudimentary at best. While the elementary level of my study of ethics may be comforting to some, it has been a source of extreme discomfort to me. I hope, however, that some of these ramblings will be of benefit to my fellow wanderers in the "bog of bioethics" (as distinct from John Bunyan's "slough of despond"). Once again, I am indebted to many who have been praying faithfully for me and for this paper and to my family for helping me and allowing me the freedom to work. Two factors have been particularly apparent as I struggled with my assigned topic. The first was great difficulty in unifying all the disparate aspects of this discussion. I have felt as if I have been working on a "quilt" with many different quilt squares and only a hazy idea how they fit together in a pattern. The lesson for me has been that the overall pattern or "big picture" may not be in full view when decisions must be made. We must do the best we can on each little "quilt square" in front of us and trust the Lord to work out the pattern. The other factor is that I have felt a sense of oppression as I worked on this project, so much so that it was often very difficult to proceed. Isaiah 41:13 helped me through a phase when I was considering abandoning the effort, "I am the Lord, your God, who takes hold of your right hand and says to you, Do not fear; I will help you."[1] Working in this area opens us to attack and oppression, there are many forces working against godly thinking and decisions, forces that would delight to see us give up trying altogether.

The field of "bioethics" is a relatively new one. The term was coined in the 1960s by Joseph Fletcher, of "situation ethics" fame. Until that time, medical ethics had been concerned mainly with the patterns of practice such as fee schedules, appropriate physician-patient relationships, etc. The major ethical debates of today were mere whispers. Historically, physicians have been a fairly homogeneous group with similar moral and ethical beliefs. For centuries, there was little debate on the contents of the Hippocratic oath as a basis for an ethical practice. Times have changed! Many of the major ethical debates of our day involve actions that are expressly prohibited by the Hippocratic oath—abortion and euthanasia, for example. For the most part, the discipline of bioethics has been removed from the arena of medicine and has been moved to philosophy, theology, and similar disciplines so completely that the average physician cannot even understand the literature or discussions about bioethical issues. Very few feel competent enough to venture an opinion or become involved in the dialogue. When I peruse bioethics publications, I am reminded of scanning the contents of my husband's ophthalmology journals. Everything seems vaguely familiar as if I *ought* to be able to understand it, but on closer examination, I am lost. It is my suspicion that both ophthalmologists and bioethicists make things purposely complicated to keep the rest of us out of their hair! I thought it prudent, therefore, to include a brief summary of the major tenets of both principle-based bioethics and the "ethic of caring."

One of the standard textbooks of principle-based biomedical ethics is *Principles of Biomedical Ethics* by Beauchamp and Childress. I have compiled some excerpts of this text in order to provide a basic guide for neophytes to the study of ethics. There is a popular series of books about computers with titles such as *DOS for Dummies*.[2] This section could probably safely be called *Ethics for the Uninitiated* and is reproduced in its entirety below. Think of it as a "translation guide" for use while reading *First Things* and other material in the field of ethics. Only a brief summary will appear in the main body of the paper. Beauchamp and Childress provide the following definition:

> Biomedical ethics involves obtaining relevant factual information, assessing its reliability, identifying moral problems, and mapping out alternative solutions to the problems that have been identified. This mapping entails presenting and defending reasons in support of one's factual, conceptual, and moral claims, while at the same time analyzing and assessing one's basic assumptions and commitments. Ideally one should also be able to anticipate and respond to reasonable objections that others might make to one's arguments and solutions.[3]

There are two main types of principle-based ethical theories—consequentialist and deontological. This classification was developed in this century to facilitate the comparison of ancient and modern theories. Utilitarianism is the best known consequentialist theory. The writings of David Hume (1711–1776), Jeremy Bentham (1748–1832), and John Stuart Mill (1806–1873) provide the foundation for utilitarianism. Beauchamp and Childress "use utilitarianism to refer to the moral theory that there is one and only one basic principle in ethics, the principle of utility, which asserts that we ought always to produce the greatest possible balance of value over disvalue (or the least possible balance of disvalue, if only undesirable results can be achieved)."[4] This has often been simplistically summarized by the statements, "The end justifies the means" or "We ought to promote the greatest good of the greatest number" or "What is right is what is most useful."[5] This theory actually encompasses a number of subclassifications including "act utilitarian" and "rule utilitarian." In addition, it is sometimes referred to as a "teleological" theory.

The *deontological* theory (*deon* is Greek for duty) has more diverse roots, including some religious traditions which focus on divine commands. Immanuel Kant (1734–1804) is credited with formulating the first integrated deontological theory. Although the range of deontological theories is even broader than that of the utilitarian theories, a summary statement is possible:

Deontological theories hold that some features of acts other than, or in addition to, their consequences make them right or wrong and that the grounds of right or obligation are not wholly dependent on the production of good consequences. The essence of the deontological perspective is that some actions are right (or wrong) for reasons other than their consequences.[6]

The difference between utilitarian and deontological thinking was well illustrated by Rabbi Marc Gellman in his discussion of Shel Silverstein's *The Giving Tree* which was published as part of a symposium in *First Things*. In the story, the tree gives everything she has in unsuccessful attempts to make "the boy" happy until she is reduced to a mere stump and the boy is a tired old man, having exploited her all his life. Rabbi Gellman writes:

On a philosophical level we can use the relationship of the tree and the boy as a way to remind ourselves of the very different judgments produced by utilitarian and deontological ethical systems. Judged by the results of her actions, the tree is culpable before the bar of utilitarian judgment because she produced a spoiled little snot. Judged by her motives, however, the tree remains deontologically pristine.[7]

More recently, in the late 1970s and the early 1980s, a new system of ethics, the "ethic of caring" or relational ethics, has added its voice to biomedical ethics discussions. A review article by Emily Hitchens and Lilyan Snow entitled "The Ethic of Caring: The Moral Response to Suffering,"[8] provides the basis for the discussion which follows. This "ethic of caring" is largely centred in the discipline of nursing and is based on the concept that truly ethical caring can take place only in a context in which the caregiver and the care-receiver are emotionally connected. "What caring comes down to, in the end, is what we do to nurture and support those people who matter to us."[9] "Relationship is what differentiates caring fidelity and promise-keeping from an approach based solely on principles, which tend to produce decisions made at a distance. Caring at its heart happens in the context of relationship."[10] "*Caring about* and *caring for* come together in acts of commitment: fidelity, keeping promises, going out of one's way, taking responsibility, developing competence"[11] These "acts of commitment" are differentiated from principles to be followed by the necessity of the context of a relationship. By implication, this relationship goes beyond the "therapeutic relationship" often used in a legal sense to define a commitment between a patient and a physician. The relationship spoken of by the proponents of the ethic of caring involves an emotional bond between caregiver and the care-receiver. Another factor which distinguishes the ethic of caring from principle-based ethics is an emphasis on mutuality in the caring relationship. "Because caring is relational, it includes attending to the well-being of the caregiver. This is not only for the pragmatic reason that care-giving requires good physical, emotional, and spiritual health, but because the caregiver is, as a human being, an equally deserving person."[12] This idea is also present in the authors' assertion, "The secret is that the one who cares is cared for in the doing."[13] Because the foundation is the relationship between the caregiver and the care-receiver, this type of caring must always be dependent on the context of the situation and cannot be abstracted to a refined set of principles with "caring" as their focus. "What to do depends on the persons, on their relationship, in the context."[14] "*Knowledge, patience, honesty, trust, humility, hope,* and *courage*" are the aspects of caring identified by Barbara Carper in a review of the caring literature published in 1979.[15] Other authors have defined the qualities of caring as "*knowing* the patient, *being with* another in an engaged manner, *doing for* patients what they cannot do for themselves, and *enabling* patients to do what they need for their own health."[16] In the paper under discussion, the authors used these qualities as guidelines in their examination of accounts of Civil War nurses in the United States. This was the era in which the discipline of modern nursing was born and these war experiences were seminal in its formation.

> Caring is ethical in that it is the right thing to do in the circumstances. Louisa May Alcott showed this ethic in action when she was nursing at Union Hotel Hospital in Georgetown:

> The next night, as I went my rounds with Dr. P., I happened to ask which man in the room probably suffered most; and, to my great surprise he glanced at John. . . . "He won't last more than a day or two, at fur-

thest . . . you'd better tell him so before long; [women have a way of doing such things comfortably, so I leave it to you . . . .]" It was an easy thing for Dr. P. to say: "Tell him he must die," but a cruelly hard thing to do. . . . A few minutes later . . . I saw John sitting erect, with no one to support him, while the surgeon dressed his back . . . [he] looked lonely and forsaken just then, as he sat with bent head, hands folded on his knee, and no outward sign of suffering, till, looking nearer, I saw great tears roll down and drop upon the floor. . . . My heart opened wide and took him in, as, gathering the bent head in my arms, as freely as if he had been a little child, I said, "Let me help you bear it, John." Never, on any human countenance, have I seen so swift and beautiful a look of gratitude, surprise and comfort, as that which answered me more eloquently than the whispered—"Thank you, ma'am, this is right good: this is what I wanted!" "Then why did you not ask for it before?" "I didn't want to be a trouble; you seemed so busy, and I could manage to get along alone." "You shall not want it any more, John."[17]

This same emphasis on the relational aspect of caring can also be applied to the health care community as a whole with the emphasis on relational aspects of working together in the delivery of health care.

Although the ethic of caring has much to commend it, several problems become evident. The relationists cannot "generalize" to produce a set of principles for use in any circumstance. In ethical jargon this would be called a lack of "universalizability." This is a serious weakness in any theory since it cannot be applied to other situations with any degree of consistency. How can one know if one is truly "caring" by the tenets of that system if each case is tested only on its own merits and only those involved can judge the quality of the relationship? There is a definite lack of objectivity. Also, if the relationship between the caregiver and the care-receiver is paramount, what happens when their beliefs or wishes conflict? How can there be resolution in the face of irreconcilable differences if there is no recognized hierarchy of principles? Does it mean, in our age of radical autonomy, that, if at all possible, the caregiver should provide exactly what the care-receiver perceives he needs? What if a patient in the terminal phase of an illness is completely convinced that he should be assisted in ending his life at a time of his own choosing? Under the ethic of caring, would the caregiver be ethically obligated to assist even if he disagreed with the patient's decision on moral grounds or felt that depression might be clouding the patient's judgment? While it is true that the relationship between caregiver and care-receiver can usually be mutually edifying, this is not always possible. If caregivers and care-receivers are "equally deserving" in the ethic of caring, what happens if mutuality is not possible or if the urgent needs of the patient far outweigh those of the caregiver? Examples of this would be a comatose terminally ill person needing total care or a patient in full cardiac arrest. Is the nurse who attends to the physical needs of the comatose patient prevented from ethical caring because there can be no mutual emotional bond between them? Is the physician who defibrillates a patient in a cardiac arrest not caring for the patient in an ethical way? If the physician never has any personal emotional connection with this patient, is the defibrillation disqualified as caring? Another area of difficulty for this theory is in public health issues. A public health official will never have a personal relationship with every person in his jurisdiction but he is still expected to make wise and ethical choices concerning the delivery of health care in his region. To say he cannot "care" for the people there because he cannot have a personal relationship with each of them is simplistic and naive. For example, much tangible good has been done for many people through the proper introduction of adequate water and sanitation facilities and the institution of immunization programs. "Caring" for children in general enough to work hard to develop safe and effective vaccines and the programs which make them accessible would still qualify as "care" to me even though few, if any, on-going personal relationships are involved. It should be noted, however, that many of those involved in research and public health initiatives are spurred on by relationships with patients which serve as "prototypes" for all the other "potential" relationships. Numerous medical advances began when a health care worker said, "Enough! Things should not have to be this way!" Dr. Cicely Saunders caught her vision for the modern

Hospice movement from comments made to her by one of her dying patients. Who could deny that millions of people around the world have received infinitely better care in their final days due to her efforts and inspiration? Would this not qualify as caring? It is evident that principle-based ethics and the ethic of caring have very different perspectives on what the general thrust of caring for a patient should involve.

Precisely what is caring? It would be wise to clarify the definition and the connotations of the term. Insights into the meaning of "care" are revealed in the examination of its linguistic origins. In English, the word "care" has its roots in the Middle English and Anglo-Saxon words *caru* or *cearu*, meaning sorrow, which are akin to the Gothic word *kara* and the German root *kar-*. There is also a probable link to the Indo-European root *gar-* which means "to cry out."[18] The origins of the word involve sorrow or worry and that connotation remains one of the meanings for the word "care." In the context of this paper, however, we shall use the meaning which connotes "to take charge of; look after; provide for; watch over; or attend to."[19]

It is not enough simply to define care, we must delineate the context in which it can fully express the meaning we assign to it. What does it mean to care for a patient? Stanley Hauerwas notes that the term "care" can be used in two contexts. "We sometimes use 'care' to indicate an attitude, feeling, or state of mind about a person or state of circumstance—'I really care for Judy.'" He also points out that "'to care' may denote a stronger intention 'to pay particular attention to.'" Hauerwas continues, "'Care' is also used in a manner that does not involve any attitude, but rather is a correlative to someone's having a certain skill. For example, we say that a mechanic cares for our car not because he likes our car, but because he possesses a technical ability that is necessary to be able to repair a car." He concludes, "The reason 'care' seems so appropriate to medical and health-related activities is that these activities involve both senses of care."[20]

Hauerwas quotes Edmund Pellegrino who asserts,

> that the physician must "have some understanding of what sickness means to another person, together with a readiness to help and to see the situation as the patient does. Compassion demands that the physician be so

disposed that his every action and word will be rooted
in respect for the person he is serving."[21]

He also reminds us that while empathy is very important, "it cannot
be forgotten that competent care is equally important . . . good
medicine should combine both."[22] Hauerwas also addresses the confusion in our culture between caring and curing. He includes Paul
Ramsey's thoughts and adds his own comments, "'Care never ceases;
yet care, never ceasing, has no duty to do the impossible or the useless.' Ramsey, therefore, seems to indicate that the 'care' incumbent
on doctors does not involve simply their medical skills, but the
moral skill to be present with those who are suffering."[23] It is interesting to note that "being present with those who are suffering" is
one of the major themes of the ethic of caring and the emphasis on
physicians being competent in their medical skills is an important
tenet of principle-based ethics.

Alastair V. Campbell tackles the subject of "Caring and Being
Cared For" in *On Moral Medicine* and adds several valuable insights.
He draws on the work of William F. May in his observations.

> May describes covenant and contract as "first cousins,"
> but goes on to argue that although they have material
> similarities, they differ radically *in spirit*. Contracts de-
> fine a precise set of relationships, and, if these are cor-
> rectly observed, then the contractual obligation is fully
> discharged. But covenants "have a gratuitous, growing
> edge to them that nourishes rather than limits relation-
> ships."[24]

He cautions against the automatic acceptance of the covenant model
of care, "The notion of contract, with its emphasis on mutual advantage, equal obligation, and clearly specified criteria for breach of
agreement, has much to commend it. A contractual approach can
protect the clients of professionals against paternalism and exploitation."[25] Contracts also serve to remind those seeking care that they
have certain responsibilities associated with their care. He seems to
advocate a professional relationship that has some aspects of both
covenant and contract. He identifies some of the pitfalls of reciproc-
ity in the caring relationship and addresses them. "Unless we recognize the element of personal need leading people into professional
caring, we shall fail to see how damaging some forms of over-

commitment can be." And, "The *need* to be helpful becomes an insistent *demand* to be perpetually rescuing people . . . the truly needy person in some helping relationships may well be the helper."[26] The introduction of grace into the caring relationship allows both the caregiver and care-receiver to benefit.

> We feel cared for when *our* need is recognized and when the help which is offered does not overwhelm us but gently restores our strength at a pace which allows us to feel part of the movement to recovery. . . . Graceful care refers to something which is not offered by anxious people trying to earn love, but by sensitive people who release us from bonds of our own making in spontaneous and often surprising ways.[27]

Campbell maintains that graceful care is often mediated through appropriate bodily expressions of care, especially touching, which may hearken back to our first caring relationship, the relationship with our own mother. He relates the story in Luke 7:36-50 about the "sinful woman" who anoints Jesus' feet and dries them with her hair and comments on Jesus' response, "He gives care by receiving care and does so in a graceful bodily way."[28] When both the caregiver and the care-receiver administer grace, the caring relationship can be healing for both. An example of this in my own life was when my sister and I gave our mother a final bath in her bed shortly before she died at home. We were able to make her physically more comfortable for a few hours, but her grateful acceptance of our ministrations continues to have a healing effect in our lives, more than ten years after the event.

In summary, we have seen care described as both an attitude and a technical ability, both of which are important for proper medical care. Respect for the person who is the patient and the moral skill to be present with him through suffering are also important. Both contract and covenant models for the physician-patient relationship were discussed with the preferred arrangement combining aspects of both. A caution was issued to avoid care based on the needs of the caregiver. And finally, care that is gracefully given and received, often accompanied by appropriate physical expressions, may provide therapeutic benefits to everyone involved. John Patrick cautions us to remember that "care" can be a "weasel word," like "health" or "values," and that it must be defined accurately and precisely and interpreted with extreme caution in other publications and contexts.

Can we as Christians contribute a unique perspective to this discussion about care? Definitely. Affirming that God is the ultimate caregiver, I propose that he is the complete fulfilment of all the requirements for *all* models of care. God is a utilitarian because he wants the highest good for each of us and for all of society. This highest good, however, is our eternal good and therefore conforms completely to his holy character and principles and thus he meets all the criteria for being a deontologist. His very nature is one of caring deeply for individuals as he seeks to deepen his personal relationships with them. He therefore fulfils all the requirements for the relationists. John Patrick calls God a "utilitarian deontologist who cares"—what a mouthful! In addition, from the principle-based perspective: he is omniscient, and therefore has no limitations in his knowledge of the past, the present, or the future (Job 38:1–42:6; Mt 11:21); omnipotent, and thus has unlimited resources (Psalm 93:1; Rev 19:6); completely loving by nature and in his actions (Is 54:10; Rom 8:31-32, 38-39); never changes (Jas 1:17; Rev 4:8); and is holy (Ex 15:11; 1 Jn 1:5). On the relational side, he has an intimate knowledge and deep, sacrificial, unconditional love for every individual who has ever lived or will ever live on the face of the earth (Jn 3:16 and Ps 139). Furthermore, he is a willing caregiver. Peter encourages his readers, "Cast all your anxiety on him because he cares for you" (1 Pet 5:7). In addition, God has the same care and concern for all his creation (Ps 24:1-2; Mt 10:29-30).

Jesus, too, is the embodiment of both principles and caring. In the first chapter of the gospel of John, we learn that Jesus is our *Logos* and in him, "the Word became flesh and made his dwelling among us . . . full of grace and truth" (v. 14). The "Word" and the "truth" referred to here encompass the entire character of God and all his precepts. Hebrews puts it this way: "In the past God spoke to our forefathers through the prophets at many times and in various ways, but in these last days he has spoken to us by his Son" (Heb 1:1-2). The "flesh" and "grace" in this passage remind us that Jesus is also our *Emmanuel,* God *with* us. In the incarnation we see the ultimate in caring relationships—God becoming a human being! This certainly qualifies under all the criteria in the ethic of caring.

There is a similar fulfilment of both types of caring in the person of the Holy Spirit. His name in Greek, *Paraklete*, means "comforter" or "one who comes along side." And in John 14:16-17 Jesus promises his disciples, "And I will ask the Father, and he will give you another Counsellor to be with you forever—the Spirit of truth," and later, "the Counsellor, the Holy Spirit, whom the Father will send in my name, will teach you all things and will remind you of everything I have said to you" (Jn 14:26).

It is clear that all three members of the trinity have all the qualities desired by both the principle-based and relational systems. Their infinite, perfect natures enable them to be perfect caregivers. Furthermore, the relationships within the godhead provide the model for our community caring. The Father, Son, and Holy Spirit manifest perfect unity and harmony but not uniformity. Being created "in his image"—*imago Dei*—gives our community life the potential to reflect this unity.

A further glimpse into ideal caring relationships can be seen in Genesis where God placed Adam and Eve in the garden of Eden and cared for them there. From the report in Genesis 3:8 of the Lord walking in the garden in the cool of the day, it seems that they even had fellowship with God face to face. Their sin ended that familiar relationship with God and set them to work in an imperfect world, at a greater distance from God. In Eden there had been no dilemmas. There *were* choices to be made, but before the Fall, dilemmas did not exist. There would have been no instances when it was impossible to be completely right. Today very few of the decisions we make will have totally positive results. We are often caught in situations in which we are trying to make the least harmful choice, based upon either our hierarchy of principles or the context of our relationships. The good news is that Jesus Christ has paid the price for that poor choice in Eden. Paul writes to the Romans,

> For if, by the trespass of the one man [Adam], death reigned through that one man, how much more will those who receive God's abundant provision of grace and of the gift of righteousness reign in life through the one man, Jesus Christ. Consequently, just as the result of one trespass was condemnation for all men, so also the result of one act of righteousness was justification

that brings life for all men. For just as through the
disobedience of the one man the many were made sinners, so also through the obedience of the one man the
many will be made righteous. Rom 5:17-19

Through Jesus' death and resurrection, it is possible for our relationship with the Father to be restored. It is this hope that calls us to
worship with Robert Herrick in his poem, "His Savior's Words, Going to the Cross":

Ah! Sion's Daughters, do not fear
    The Cross, the Cords, the Nails, the Spear,
    The Myrrh, the Gall, the Vinegar:
For Christ, your loving Savior, hath
    Drunk up the wine of God's fierce wrath;
    Only there's left a little froth,
Less for taste, than for to show,
    What bitter cups had been your due,
    Had He not drank them up for you.[29]

Even though we are deeply grateful for the finished work of
Christ on the cross, it is also true that we begin from a position of
being finite and living in a fallen world. But it is true as well that as
Christians the Holy Spirit indwells us and his power is available to
us. God has promised wisdom when needed, "If any of you lacks
wisdom, he should ask God, who gives generously to all without
finding fault, and it will be given to him" (Jas 1:5). And Jesus said, "I
tell you the truth, anyone who has faith in me will do what I have
been doing. He will do even greater things than these, because I am
going to the Father" (Jn 14:12). This is especially exciting in light of
Jesus' own description of his ministry when he quoted from the
prophet Isaiah, "The Spirit of the Lord is on me, because he has
anointed me to preach good news to the poor. He has sent me to
proclaim freedom for the prisoners and recovery of sight for the
blind, to release the oppressed, to proclaim the year of the Lord's
favour," and finished with, "Today this scripture is fulfilled in your
hearing" (Lk 4:18-19, 21). And by virtue of this restored relationship
and the empowering of the Holy Spirit, we are able to recapture the
spirit of Eden. Alastair V. Campbell notes, "The consistent attention
which a humane doctor offers a damaged fellow human being reveals a vision behind the Cross to a young wood in a green corner of

Eden."[30] Eden was perfect because it was based completely on love; it was also able to be based completely on love because it was perfect! Sin and imperfection entered the world and suddenly "rights" became necessary.[31] We can no longer depend on our own or anyone else's motivation to be based solely on love. There is a far greater likelihood that we will be motivated by self-interest. Although rights are imperative for any justice to prevail in our fallen world, they are really just "necessary evils" that protect us from one another, personally and as groups. Rather than taking pride that we have an extensive system of rights, we should be mourning the need for rights in the first place! If everyone in the world followed Paul's advice to the Philippians, rights would be superfluous, "Do nothing out of selfish ambition or vain conceit, but in humility consider others better than yourselves. Each of you should look not only to your own interests, but also to the interests of others" (Phil 2:3-4).

Jesus illustrates his practical definition of caring in the parable of the good Samaritan:

> On one occasion an expert in the law stood up to test Jesus. "Teacher," he asked, "what must I do to inherit eternal life?"
>
> "What is written in the Law?" he replied. "How do you read it?"
>
> He answered: "'Love the Lord your God with all your heart and with all your soul and with all your strength and with all your mind'; and, 'Love your neighbour as yourself.'"
>
> "You have answered correctly," Jesus replied. "Do this and you will live."
>
> But he wanted to justify himself, so he asked Jesus, "And who is my neighbour?"
>
> In reply Jesus said: "A man was going down from Jerusalem to Jericho, when he fell into the hands of robbers. They stripped him of his clothes, beat him and went away, leaving him half dead. A priest happened to be going down the same road, and when he saw the man, he passed by on the other side. So too, a Levite, when he came to the place and saw him, passed by on the other side. But a Samaritan, as he travelled, came

where the man was; and when he saw him, he took pity on him. He went to him and bandaged his wounds, pouring on oil and wine. Then he put the man on his own donkey, took him to an inn and took care of him. The next day he took out two silver coins and gave them to the innkeeper. 'Look after him,' he said, 'and when I return, I will reimburse you for any extra expense you may have.'

"Which of these three do you think was a neighbour to the man who fell into the hands of robbers?"

The expert of the law replied, "The one who had mercy on him."

Jesus told him, "Go and do likewise." (Lk 10:25-37)

In this parable, Jesus identifies three potential helpers for the robbed man: a priest; a Levite, an assistant to the priests who was a descendant of Levi but not Aaron; and the Samaritan, despised by the Jews because he was of mixed race being descended from Gentiles and the Israelites left behind when the Northern kingdom of Israel fell to the Assyrians. It behoves us to remember that the priest and the Levite were well respected religious leaders in Jesus' day. The Samaritan, however, would have had religious beliefs that were heretical to the Jews. Jesus' point was not to commend the Samaritan's religious views, but rather to illustrate that the practical application of the two greatest commandments is found in how we treat our neighbours. Jesus was much more impressed with the Samaritan's heart and actions (his "orthopraxy") than with the probable orthodoxy of the priest and the Levite.[32] Like the priest, the Levite, and the lawyer who asked the question, we, too, are most comfortable in the realm of knowledge and theory. Dr. J. I. Packer once commented that God delights in giving practical answers to theoretical questions—"You're concerned about who is going to heaven? Good! So am I, go tell everyone about me!" This ends the useless debates about whether those who have never heard the gospel will or will not be saved. Jesus' response to the lawyer is another instance of a practical answer to a theoretical question—"You want to know who your neighbour is? I'll tell you—it is the person who is near you whose needs you have the ability to meet." Period. Not an answer to the question, "Who is my neighbour so I can figure out whose needs

I may ignore?" In addition to his desire to test Jesus, this self-justifying attitude seems to be at the heart of the lawyer's question. In other words, "How can I get 'off the hook' as much as possible?" Jesus puts us firmly back "on the hook" in our responsibility to care for those around us.

As followers of Christ, how *do* we go about caring? *Compassion* is a profound book by Donald P. McNeill, Douglas A. Morrison, and Henri J. M. Nouwen which explores this subject. I am indebted to them for many of the insights in the remainder of this paper. It seems that there are two main things we must do in order to care as Jesus calls us to care. The first is to be empty and the second is to allow him to fill us. Emptying ourselves starts with our attitude matching Jesus' attitude. Paul reminded the Philippians, "*Your attitude should be the same as that of Christ Jesus:* Who, being in very nature God, did not consider equality with God something to be grasped, but made himself nothing, taking the very nature of a servant, being made in human likeness. And being found in appearance as a man, he humbled himself and became obedient to death—even death on a cross!" (Phil 2:5-8, emphasis mine). It is when we accept our own inability to care in our own strength and our utter dependence on his enabling, that we begin to be useful to God. Jesus reminds us of this reality in John 15:4-5, "No branch can bear fruit by itself; it must remain in the vine. Neither can you bear fruit unless you remain in me. I am the vine; you are the branches. If a man remains in me and I in him, he will bear much fruit; apart from me you can do nothing." In the Sermon on the Mount, Jesus emphasizes the paramount importance of this heart attitude, "Blessed are the poor in spirit, for theirs is the kingdom of heaven" (Mt 5:3). *Ptochos*, the Greek word translated *poor*, means *utterly destitute and totally incapable of helping one's self.* Jesus is saying that people who acknowledge their poverty of spirit are *blessed* or *spiritually prosperous*. In Matthew 5:20 he continues, "Unless your righteousness surpasses that of the Pharisees and the teachers of the law, you will certainly not enter the kingdom of heaven." Like the Pharisees and teachers we want a set of rules, a system of ethics, to follow. God wants our actions to be the obedient fruit of a changed heart. Paul understood that our usefulness is rooted in our weakness. He wrote to the Corinthians, "But we have this treasure in jars of clay to show that this all-surpassing power is from God and not from us" (2 Cor 4:7). He also told them of the Lord's response when he had asked for his "thorn in the flesh" to be removed, "My grace is sufficient for you, for my power is made perfect in weakness" (2 Cor 12:9). Just how *can* this self-emptying become a reality in our lives? I think there will be both personal and corporate applications. These will be different for each person, but there are some areas where physicians will tend to have common struggles in moving from principle to practice. So, how do we "remain in the vine?" How do we allow his glory to shine through? If God is the source of our power and wisdom, we must follow his direction. It is interesting to note that the word for obedience is derived from the Latin word *audire*, meaning "to listen." Obedience is impossible without listening to God. This means sacrificing our personal agendas to set time aside for Scripture study, contemplation, and prayer, just as Jesus did. Our biggest deterrent for this is busyness and over-commitment. In his book, *Margin*,[33] physician Richard Swenson documents the exponential rise in the availability of information and the rate of cultural change. In the Western world, our response has been to increase the complexity and pace of our lives in a vain effort to "keep up." By the time we realise the impossibility of this task, we are almost irrevocably entangled in a high pressure lifestyle with little or no discretionary time. Swenson visualizes our lives as printed pages and says that we have filled the pages all the way to the edges—our lives are "marginless." This has many detrimental effects, but one major result is that we leave no time or energy to put at the Lord's disposal. If every minute of every day is double-booked and we are chronically exhausted and cranky, how can we ever hope to be available to the Lord when he could use some *unscheduled* or *sustained* human assistance? We are too busy, often with good and worthy pursuits, to notice our neighbours. We end up "passing by on the other side" because we allow the "good" in our lives to crowd out the "best." The first step toward more meaningful caring relationships may be to slow down and simplify, to leave room for the focus to shift away from ourselves to others.

> To pay attention to others with the desire to make them
> the center and to make their interests our own is a real
> form of self-emptying, since to be able to receive others

into our intimate inner space we must be empty. That is why listening is so difficult. It means our moving away from the center of attention and inviting others into that space. . . . The simple experience of being valuable and important to someone else has a tremendous rec-reative power.[34]

And it takes time. We often complain about being too busy, but in reality many of us enjoy the feeling of being indispensable and the image that we are dedicated and over-worked. Many physicians have also fallen into the ever-tightening grasp of materialism. In doing so they bind themselves firmly to a frenetic pace of life as government cutbacks result in the necessity to work longer for the same remu-neration. We need to take a long, hard look at ourselves in light of Jesus' ministry, noting that God himself took time to rest, pray, re-flect, and commune with loved ones without attempting to meet every need around him. His life was completely consistent with his name, *Jehovah Shalom*—the God of peace with order. I must admit that in regard to over-commitment I am the "chief of sinners." A substantial part of this paper was completed after midnight and household tasks were left undone for weeks while I concentrated on writing. How much margin can there be in my own life when just doing the laundry is a crisis? Over-commitment is a sin, not an ex-cuse for self-pity. I do not have any facile solutions, but this problem is a source of pain for me and my family and I know that I need to go before the Lord in prayerful consideration about this issue, per-haps you do, too. Slowing the whirling dervish of a marginless life to allow time and energy for a life of compassion is not easy or simple. This, too, is only possible as a gift of his grace. "We need to be re-minded continuously that compassion is not conquered but given, not the outcome of our hard work but the fruit of God's grace."[35]

Another way we empty ourselves is by discarding our personal, romantic ideas about what it means to serve God. This frees us to go where and when we are called, on his terms. Like the proverbial story of well-intentioned citizens forcing an elderly lady to cross a street she had not intended to cross, our efforts at caring and com-passion can go terribly wrong unless we rely on God's wisdom in-stead of our own. Jesus followed his Father's way of sacrifice and ser-vanthood. "Jesus' whole life and mission involve accepting power-

lessness and revealing in this powerlessness the limitlessness of
God's love. Here we see what compassion means. It is not a bending
toward the underprivileged from a privileged position; it is not a
reaching out from on high to those who are less fortunate below; it
is not a gesture of sympathy or pity for those who fail to make it in
the upward pull. On the contrary, compassion means going directly
to those people and places where suffering is most acute and building a home there."[36] This is powerful. Jesus did not reach *down* to us
from on high and pull us up to his level but he came to us, emptying
himself to serve in humility. Frequently, we choose our opportunities for "service" based upon sentimentality, paternalism, or even
our own needs.

> We often think that service means to give something to
> others, to tell them how to speak, act, or behave; but
> now it appears that above all else, real, humble service
> is helping our neighbors discover that they possess great
> but often hidden talents that can enable them to do
> even more for us than we can do for them. By revealing
> the unique gifts of the other, we learn to empty our-
> selves. Self-emptying does not ask of us to engage our-
> selves in some form of self-castigation or self-scrutiny,
> but to pay attention to others in such a way that they
> begin to recognize their own value.[37]

A compelling example of this is the interaction Jesus had with the
woman at the well in John chapter four. Their relationship began as
he graciously acknowledged his own need and asked her, a social
outcast, for a drink of water. In their candid interchange she saw her
own life with blinding clarity but Jesus did not leave her desolate.
She was the first person to whom he revealed that he was the promised Messiah, transforming her life into one of hope. We, too, can
minister his grace, especially to those who are suffering, by emptying
ourselves, going to meet them, staying with them in their pain, and
never failing to offer hope.

Being empty, and therefore available for the Lord to care
through us, also has a place in our corporate life as the body of
Christ. Nouwen et al. stress that the Christian community is
uniquely suited to be the best mediator between individual believers
and the world's needs, which often overwhelm and paralyse us. "In

community, we are no longer a mass of helpless individuals, but are transformed into one people of God . . . in the way we live and work together, God's compassion becomes present in the midst of a broken world."[38] Our ability to serve (care) effectively has its foundation in our community life.

> Servanthood too is a quality of the community. . . . As individuals we cannot be everything to everyone, but as a community we can indeed serve a great variety of needs. Moreover, by the constant support and encouragement of the community we find it possible to remain faithful to our commitment to service. Finally, we must recognize that obedience, as an attentive listening to the Father, is very much a communal vocation. It is precisely by constant prayer and meditation that the community remains alert and open to the needs of the world.[39]

"In the intimacy of prayer, God reveals himself to us as the God who loves all the members of the human family just as personally and uniquely as he loves us. Therefore a growing intimacy with God deepens our sense of responsibility for others. . . . Compassionate prayer is a mark of the Christian community."[40] This is not perfunctory prayer, an afterthought to ask the Lord's blessing on endeavours already planned. It is sustained, active patience as represented by the word *hypomone*, which is also translated *endurance*, *perseverance*, and *fortitude*.[41] The connection of the Lord's supper with our communal work of compassion is particularly meaningful:

> In the breaking of bread together, we give the clearest testimony to the communal character of our prayers. . . . [It] is the celebration, the making present, of Christ's story as well as our own. In the taking, blessing, breaking, and giving of the bread, the mystery of Christ's life is expressed in the most succinct way. The Father took his only Son and sent him into the world so that through him the world might be saved (Jn 3:17). At the river Jordan and on Mount Tabor he blessed him with the words, "This is my Son, the Beloved, my favor rests on him . . . listen to him" (Mt 3:17, 17:5). The blessed one was broken on a cross, "pierced

through for our faults, crushed for our sins" (Is 53:5). But through his death he gives himself to us as our food, thus fulfilling the words he spoke to his disciples at the last supper, "This is my body which will be given for you" (Lk 22:19). It is in this life that is taken, blessed, broken, and given that Jesus Christ wants to make us participants.[42]

A case I was involved in several years ago in Halifax, Nova Scotia, illustrates many of the concepts under discussion. A beautiful, talented, athletic, nineteen-year-old young woman lost her long battle with a sarcoma in her leg. She was able to be cared for in her own room, in her own home because of the combined efforts of her family, her family physician, her oncologist, the visiting Palliative Care nurses, accompanied by a Palliative Care physician on occasion, her church, and her community at large. Although no one could have managed her care alone, the contributions of all these individuals made it possible for her to be relatively comfortable and to live her life with tremendous vitality. The last few hours of her life were difficult, however. The cancer had invaded her lungs to such an extent that breathing suddenly became nearly impossible. In response to an urgent, 5 A.M. phone call from her mother, I met them in the emergency department of the hospital. After several unsuccessful interventions, the patient asked us to stop further treatment attempts, and died in her mother's arms a few moments later. What possible comfort could there be for these bereaved parents? The patient and her family were all strong Christians, but the pain of her loss was still overwhelming. And yet, somehow by the grace of God, I was able to stand with them in their pain that morning and minister his peace that passes understanding. How do I know this? Because four months later, after a particularly difficult time in my own life, I arrived at the hospital to find a card and a large box from this patient's mother. Inside were two beautiful stuffed rabbits that she had made. The card expressed deep gratitude for all that we had done to assist them through their difficult time. The love shown to me through this generous gift "restored my soul." Today, those rabbits reside on my bedside table to remind me of a courageous young woman, her mother's gift of compassion, the precious brevity of life, and the great privilege it is to comfort fellow travellers and *be comforted* in

return. In this incident in my own life, there was a definite integration of principles and relational caring, and it was both excruciating
and magnificent.

One piece of the pattern for this paper was in place from an
early stage: Revelation 21:3-5 was to be the conclusion. These verses
describing the new Jerusalem strike me as being particularly meaningful to the health care community.

> And I heard a loud voice from the throne saying, "Now
> the dwelling of God is with men, and he will live with
> them. They will be his people, and God himself will be
> with them and be their God. He will wipe away every
> tear from their eyes. There will be no more death or
> mourning or crying or pain, for the old order of things
> has passed away." He who was seated on the throne
> said, "I am making everything new!" Then he said,
> "Write this down, for these words are trustworthy and
> true."

It is fitting that Henri Nouwen and friends also chose this passage as
their concluding Scripture. They offered these insights:

> In the new city, God will live among us, but each time
> two or three gather in the name of Jesus he is already in
> our midst. In the new city, all tears will be wiped away,
> but each time people eat bread and drink wine in his
> memory, smiles appear on strained faces. In the new
> city, the whole creation will be made new, but each time
> prison walls are broken down, poverty is dispelled, and
> wounds are carefully attended, the old earth is already
> giving way to the new. Through compassionate action,
> the old is not just old anymore and pain not just pain
> any longer. Although we are still waiting in expectation,
> the first signs of the new earth and the new heaven,
> which have been promised to us and for which we
> hope, are already visible in the community of faith
> where the compassionate God reveals himself. This is
> the foundation of our faith, the basis of our hope, the
> source of our love.[43]

Appendix: A Brief Synopsis of Principle-based Ethics Excerpted from Beauchamp and Childress

Although this part of the discussion may seem dry and academic in the extreme, it is provided with the sincere hope that it will be a sort of "travellers' dictionary" for colleagues embarking on reading and discussions in the field of biomedical ethics.

Beauchamp and Childress provide the following definition:

> Biomedical ethics involves obtaining relevant factual information, assessing its reliability, identifying moral problems, and mapping out alternative solutions to the problems that have been identified. This mapping entails presenting and defending reasons in support of one's factual, conceptual, and moral claims, while at the same time analyzing and assessing one's basic assumptions and commitments. Ideally one should also be able to anticipate and respond to reasonable objections that others might make to one's arguments and solutions.[44]

They describe the hierarchy of ethical thought as: "Particular judgments are justified by moral rules, which in turn are justified by principles, which ultimately are defended by an ethical theory."[45] They further define their terms in the following section: "As we analyze them, *rules* are more specific to contexts and more restricted in scope. A simple example of a rule is "It is wrong to lie to a patient." *Principles* are more general and fundamental than moral rules and serve to justify the rules. For example, a principle of respect for autonomy may support several moral rules of the form 'It is wrong to lie.' Finally, *theories* are integrated bodies of principles and rules and may include mediating rules that govern choices in cases of conflicts."[46] *Action-guides* is a general term used by Beauchamp and Childress which most often replaces *principles* or *rules* but may also refer to theories.

In their more detailed discussion of the structure of the study of ethics, they offer the following general comments:

> *Ethics* is a generic term for several ways of examining the moral life. Some approaches to ethics are normative, others descriptive. . . . The field of inquiry that attempts to answer the question "Which action-guides are worthy of moral acceptance and for what reasons?" may

> be called *general normative ethics.* . . . The attempts to apply these action-guides to different moral problems can be labeled *applied normative ethics.* . . . There are at least two non-normative approaches to ethics. First, *descriptive ethics* is the factual investigation of moral behavior and beliefs. It studies not what people ought to do but how they reason and act. . . . Second, *metaethics* involves analysis of the language, concepts, thought, and objects of ethics. For example, it studies the meanings of crucial ethical terms such as *right, obligation, virtue,* and *responsibility,* as well as the logic and patterns of moral reasoning and justification.[47]

Clinical biomedical ethics is a division of applied normative ethics. In short, normative ethics take a moral position while non-normative ethics do not take a moral position.

There are two main types of ethical theories, *consequentialist* and *deontological.* This classification was developed in this century to facilitate the comparison of ancient and modern theories. *Utilitarianism* is the best known consequentialist theory. The writings of David Hume (1711–1776), Jeremy Bentham (1748–1832), and John Stuart Mill (1806–1873) provide the foundation for utilitarianism. Beauchamp and Childress "use *utilitarianism* to refer to the moral theory that there is one and only one basic principle in ethics, the principle of utility, which asserts that we ought always to produce the greatest possible balance of value over disvalue (or the least possible balance of disvalue, if only undesirable results can be achieved)."[48] This has often been simplistically summarized by the statements, "The end justifies the means" or "We ought to promote the greatest good of the greatest number" or "What is right is what is most useful."[49] This theory is actually encompasses a number of subclassifications including "act utilitarian" and "rule utilitarian." In addition, it is sometimes referred to as a "teleological" theory.

The *deontological* theory (*deon* is Greek for duty) has more diverse roots, including some religious traditions which focus on divine commands. Immanuel Kant (1734–1804) is credited with formulating the first integrated deontological theory. Although the range of deontological theories is even more diverse than that of the utilitarian theories, a summary statement is possible:

Deontological theories hold that some features of acts other than, or in addition to, their consequences make them right or wrong and that the grounds of right or obligation are not wholly dependent on the production of good consequences. The essence of the deontological perspective is that some actions are right (or wrong) for reasons other than their consequences.[50]

The difference between utilitarian and deontological thinking was well illustrated by Rabbi Marc Gellman in his discussion of Shel Silverstein's *The Giving Tree* which was published as part of a symposium in *First Things*. In the story, the tree gives everything she has in unsuccessful attempts to make "the boy" happy until she is reduced to a mere stump and the boy is a tired old man, having exploited her all his life. Rabbi Gellman writes:

On a philosophical level we can use the relationship of the tree and the boy as a way to remind ourselves of the very different judgments produced by utilitarian and deontological ethical systems. Judged by the results of her actions, the tree is culpable before the bar of utilitarian judgment because she produced a spoiled little snot. Judged by her motives, however, the tree remains deontologically pristine."[51]

Now that we have a primitive understanding of the foundations of the major theories within principle-based ethics, it is time to determine just what these theories would identify as "good care." Here is a list of some of the major ethical precepts common to all "principle-based" ethical theories. They are given in point form to aid in clarity and simplicity.[52]

1. *Respect for Persons:* The duty to respect the self-determination and choices of autonomous persons, as well as to protect persons with diminished autonomy, e.g., young children, mentally retarded persons, and those with other mental impairments.

2. *Informed Consent:* The obligation to ensure the adequate disclosure and comprehension by patients of medical information related to medical decision making surrounding their care and their voluntary, competent consent to medical decisions and agreements.

3. *Beneficence*: The obligation to secure the well-being of persons by acting positively on their behalf and, moreover, to maximize the benefits that can be obtained.

4. *Non-maleficence*: The obligation to minimize the harm to persons and, wherever possible, to remove the causes of harm altogether.

5. *Proportionality*: The duty, when taking actions involving risks of harm, to so balance risks and benefits that actions have the greatest chance to result in the least harm and the most benefit to persons directly involved.

6. *Justice*: The obligation to distribute benefits and burdens fairly, to treat equals equally, and to give reasons for differential treatment based on widely accepted criteria for just ways to distribute benefits and burdens.

Adherents to any of the principle-based ethical theories would agree that if all of these precepts have been followed and there were no conflicts between them, the patient would have received the proper care.

The "principle of double effect" is also an important concept in principle-based ethics.

According to this principle there is a morally relevant difference between the intended effects of a person's action and the nonintended though foreseen effects of the action. . . . The principle of double effect specifies four conditions that must be satisfied for an act with both a good and a bad effect to be justified. (1) The action itself (independent of its consequences) must not be intrinsically wrong (it must be morally good or at least morally neutral). (2) The agent must intend only the good effect and not the bad effect. The bad effect can be foreseen, tolerated, and permitted but must not be intended; it is therefore allowed but not sought. . . . (3) The bad effect must not be a means to the end of bringing about the good effect; that is, the good effect must be achieved directly by the action and not by way of the bad effect. (4) The good result must outweigh the evil permitted; that is, there must be proportionality or a favorable balance between the good and bad effects of the action.[53]

An example of this principle in action would be if giving a large dose of opioid medication in order to relieve intractable pain in a terminally ill patient *appeared* to have caused the patient to die sooner than expected. How does the principle of double effect apply in this case? (1) It is not intrinsically wrong to give a large dose of opioid medication to a terminally ill patient. (2) The only intention in giving the medication was the relief of pain, although the physician knew there was a potential for shortening the patient's life. (3) The good effect—relief of the pain—was not intended to be accomplished by killing the patient, only by giving an adequate dose of opioid medication. (4) The probable good result of relieving the pain was deemed to be worth the very minimal risk of shortening the life of a terminally ill patient.

Beauchamp and Childress also acknowledge that

broad scientific, metaphysical, or religious beliefs may underlie our interpretation of a situation, and moral debate about a particular course of action may stem not only from disagreements about the relevant moral action-guides and the facts of the case but also from disagreements about the correct scientific, metaphysical, or religious description of the situation.[54]

They also note that: "The fact that no currently available theory, whether rule utilitarian or rule deontological, adequately resolves all moral conflicts points to their incompleteness. But this incompleteness may reflect the complex and sometimes dilemmatic character of the moral life rather than inherent defects in the theories."[55] It is also true that this approach to ethics pays little attention to interpersonal relationships and can be very cold and harsh when applied.

Notes

1   Unless otherwise noted, all Scriptural quotations in this article are taken from the New International Version of the Bible, copyright the New York International Bible Society.

2   Dan Gookin, *DOS for Dummies, Windows 95 Edition* (Foster City, Calif.: IDG Books Worldwide, 1996).

3   Tom L. Beauchamp and James F. Childress, *Principles of Biomedical Ethics*, 3rd ed. (New York: Oxford University Press, 1989), 21.

[4] Ibid., 26.

[5] Ibid.

[6] Ibid., 36.

[7] Marc Gellman, "The Giving Tree: A Symposium," *First Things* 49 (January 1995): 38.

[8] Emily Hitchens and Lilyan Snow, "The Ethic of Caring: The Moral Response to Suffering," *Christian Scholar's Review* 23, no. 3 (1994): 307–17.

[9] Ibid., 307.

[10] Ibid., 308.

[11] Ibid., 308, n. 6.

[12] Ibid., 308.

[13] Ibid., 316.

[14] Ibid., 313.

[15] Ibid., 309, n. 10.

[16] Ibid., 309, n. 11.

[17] Ibid., 313.

[18] *Webster's New World Dictionary of the American Language* (Cleveland: World Publishing Co., 1962), s. v. "care."

[19] Ibid., 221.

[20] *On Moral Medicine, Theological Perspectives in Medical Ethics*, ed. Stephen E. Lammers and Allen Verhey (Grand Rapids, Mich.: William B. Eerdmans, 1989), 262.

[21] Ibid., 263.

[22] Ibid.

[23] Ibid., 265.

[24] Ibid., 267.

[25] Ibid.

[26] Ibid., 268.

[27] Ibid., 269.

[28] Ibid.

[29] Robert Atwan and Laurance Wieder, ed., *Chapters Into Verse*, vol. 2 (Oxford: Oxford University Press, 1993), 195–96.

[30] Campbell, *On Moral Medicine*, 271.

[31] Many thanks for this insight to Iain Benson, lawyer with the Centre for Renewal in Public Policy.

[32] Many thanks for this thought to H. Dale Burke, Senior Pastor of the First Evangelical Free Church of Fullerton, California.

[33] Richard A. Swenson, MD, *Margin: How to Create the Emotional, Physical, Financial, & Time Reserves You Need* (Colorado Springs, Col.: NavPress Publishing Group, 1992), 275.

34 Donald P. McNeill, Douglas A. Morrison, and Henri J. M. Nouwen, *Compassion: A Reflection on the Christian Life* (New York: Image Books, Doubleday, 1982), 81.

35 Ibid., 90.

36 Ibid., 27.

37 Ibid., 80.

38 Ibid., 56.

39 Ibid., 58.

40 Ibid., 109–10.

41 Ibid., 94.

42 Ibid., 112–13.

43 Ibid., 134–35.

44 Beauchamp, *Principles of Biomedical Ethics*, 21.

45 Ibid., 7.

46 Ibid.

47 Ibid., 9–10.

48 Ibid., 26.

49 Ibid.

50 Ibid., 36.

51 Gellman, "The Giving Tree," 38.

52 Many thanks to Ben Gibbard for this classification system.

53 Beauchamp, *Principles of Biomedical Ethics*, 127–28.

54 Ibid., 7.

55 Ibid., 46.

Sheila Rutledge Harding

Sanctity of Life, Quality of Life, and the Christian Physician

R oss is our younger son. He's nine years old. He has a very rare genetic disorder called Menkes disease which the books still say is uniformly fatal in infancy. The oldest survivor, now nineteen, was the first to be treated with an experimental drug called copper histidine. Ross has received a daily injection of copper histidine since he was four weeks old. Although this treatment has prevented the neurologic damage typical of Menkes disease, it doesn't reverse the substantial problems that these boys have with impaired energy metabolism and defective formation of connective tissues—muscles, ligaments and such.

We consider Ross to be a gift to us and the world. Other, less biased observers agree with us. He is bright, affectionate, articulate, perceptive, funny, and occasionally prophetic. In his first six years he weathered several life-threatening medical crises. On occasion, a junior paediatric trainee who knew the books, but did not yet know the boy, questioned the appropriateness of aggressive intervention for a child "who is going to be dead soon, anyway." The senior trainees simply said, "Ask us that again in two or three days, if you still think it's relevant." It has been our experience that anyone who spends time with Ross knows without a doubt that his is a life worth living, and worth fighting for. The uncertainty of his future just adds poignancy to the present. More recently, he has been consistently healthy, despite his physical limitations. Many people—doctors, nurses, pharmacists, therapists, and others—have worked very hard to enhance his quality of life, while he enriches ours.

A scientific paper is currently being written to describe four of the boys with classical Menkes disease who were started on copper histidine within the first few weeks of life. Ross is Patient 3, so we were asked to read a draft for accuracy in the description of his medical course. This scientific, ostensibly objective paper states:

> Enthusiasm about the use of this treatment . . . should be tempered by caution since the residual abnormalities may become more disabling later in life. Expectations should be especially cautious in symptomatic patients like Patient 3. . . .
>
> The treatment should still be regarded as experimental and not yet a serious alternative to early prenatal diagnosis and termination of affected pregnancies for those who regard this approach as acceptable. It is worthy of consideration for couples who cannot accept this approach.[1]

Given this attitude on the part of the experts—that the disability these boys have or may have in the future justifies the decision to abort all affected boys—Menkes disease is quickly becoming a disorder that is uniformly fatal *in utero* when the mother is a known carrier. And these experts aren't unique. Susan Massie, the mother of a haemophilic son, says:

> Doctors are left to their own prejudices. Much of what passes under the guise of medical counseling really consists only of saying no; of advising the safe way, the way of least resistance. Not long ago, I attended a medical symposium and heard a famous geneticist talk learnedly about the need for "objective" counseling in cases of genetic disease. Fine. Then he concluded his remarks with this highly subjective sentence: "I cannot imagine a family who would not *wish to avoid* the emotional and financial stress imposed upon them when a hemophiliac is born." . . .
>
> If genetic counseling is to be meaningful, then not only must those counseled be informed of the purely scientific facts, they must also be encouraged to believe in themselves, in their own capacities to live and grow. They must be counseled not only to *fear*, but to be brave enough to live with a question. . . .
>
> A child with a genetic illness is a perpetual question,

pushing us to seek answers to this dilemma of nature and God.[2]

When I started my medical training, there were a couple of things I took as givens: that medicine was an honourable profession committed to the sanctity of life; and that in my role as physician I would do all that I could on behalf of my patients to enhance their quality of life. Now, almost twenty years later, I find myself practising medicine and caring for a disabled child surrounded by a culture of death in which a concept generally referred to as Quality of Life is often used to justify violation of the principle of the Sanctity of Life. What follows are reflections on the reading I've been doing around these two ideas, sanctity and quality of life; a story; and an effort to articulate what our task as Christian physicians might be.

In a study paper for the Law Reform Commission of Canada, Keyserlingk asserts that the principle of the sanctity of life has two roots:

1. Man's dignity, worth and sanctity are from God, and not due to some quality or ability in man.
2. Life is a gift in trust, it is on loan, man does not have dominion over it.[3]

There is support for these roots in most religious traditions. Here is a sampling of what some other writers have said:

> One grasps the religious outlook upon the sanctity of human life only if he sees that this life is asserted to be surrounded by sanctity that need not be in a man; that the most dignity a man ever possesses is a dignity that is alien to him. . . . The value of a human life is ultimately grounded in the value God is placing on it.[4]

> Life does not itself create this respect. The command of God creates respect for it. When man in faith in God's Word and promise realizes how God from eternity has maintained and loved him in his little life, and what he has done for him in time, . . . he is faced by a majestic, dignified and holy fact. In human life itself he meets something superior. He is thus summoned to respect because the living God has distinguished it in this way and taken it to Himself.[5]

Man is not absolutely master of his own life and body. He has no dominion over it, but holds it in trust for God's purposes.[6]

Every human being is a unique, unrepeatable opportunity to praise God. His life is entirely an ordination, a loan, and a stewardship.[7]

These roots, taken together, lead to three assertions:

1. The sanctity of human life is not the result of the "worth" a human being may attribute to it—either to one's own life or that of others. Considerations such as "degrees of relative worth," "functional proficiency," or "pragmatic utility" . . . are in no sense appropriate yardsticks for determining or measuring sanctity of life.

2. Human life may not be taken without adequate justification, nor may human nature be radically changed.

3. The sanctity of life principle is basic to our society, and its rejection would endanger all human life.[8]

Now, is this principle of the sanctity of life in conflict with the concept of the quality of life?

The answer of course depends upon what is meant, or what meaning we give to "quality of life." What makes the question one of practical relevance and not just academic interest is that quality of life concerns are already and long have been influencing medical decisions. But what makes the question . . . [a] worrisome one for society, medicine and law is that quality of life . . . mean[s] many very different things, has no single, generally accepted meaning, and some of its connotations and the uses to which the concept is put are definitely . . . in conflict with the sanctity of life principle outlined earlier.[9]

Take, for example, this editorial from *California Medicine* in September, 1970:

The traditional Western ethic has always placed great emphasis on the intrinsic worth and equal value of every human life regardless of stage or condition. . . . This traditional ethic is still clearly dominant, but there is much to suggest that it is being eroded at its core and may eventually be abandoned. . . . There is a quite new emphasis on something which is beginning to be called the quality of life. . . . It will become necessary and acceptable to place relative rather than absolute values on such things as human lives, the use of scarce resources and the various elements which are to make up the quality of life or of living which is to be sought.[10]

I agree with Keyserlingk when he says

I [must] . . . very explicitly [part] company with the most frequently proposed meaning or connotation of quality of life in the medical . . . context—namely that it must inevitably and fundamentally involve more or less wholly subjective judgments about the relative individual or social worth, value, usefulness or equality of the lives of persons. Both proponents as well as opponents of the quality of life concept generally assume or claim that such notions are at the centre of the concept. There is little doubt that it is exactly that unqualified assumption on both sides of the argument which gives quality of life such a "bad press" and raises fears of "playing God" with human lives. If the concept is to serve [a] useful function . . . it needs rescuing as much from its proponents who claim too much for it as from its opponents who claim too little. Inasmuch as the sanctity of life principle insists that the respect and protection due to human life ought not to be based on judgments of relative worth, value or usefulness, such versions are rightly seen as opposed to and judged wanting by, the sanctity of life principle.[11]

So, can this concept of quality of life be rescued, redeemed, put to a useful purpose? I think it can, although we may wish to choose a different phrase to avoid confusion. It is useful to examine how other disciplines use this concept:

Quality of life in [environmental/social] contexts focuses on improving the quality of life for members of a society or region—better air, food, privacy, water, education, leisure, working conditions, health and so on.

>In those contexts, efforts to measure and improve the quality of life have been generally welcomed. . . . [In those] contexts the "life" being evaluated is not "John Smith's" life, but life in a particular society or region. It involves comparison . . . [However,] the things compared are not particular lives, but the "relevant environmental conditions of life" in a certain region . . . [in order to assess] their capacity to make the lives of those living in them as good as possible, or at least enable them to do so.[12]

Isn't palliative care simply the use of various strategies in patient care because of their capacity to make the lives of those cared for as good as possible? Quality of life considerations in medicine need not mean placing relative value on human lives.

>Excluded here . . . [should be] considerations such as . . . social utility, social status or relative worth [as a necessary qualification for treatment.] . . . The real question and issue raised by considerations of quality of life is not about the value of this patient's life—it is about the value of this patient's treatment.[13]

To reiterate: quality of life is not about the value of this patient's life—it is about the value of the patient's treatment. Together with our patients, we physicians make such judgments about treatment options all the time. Let us assume that Regimen A and Regimen B have identical outcomes with respect to the control or cure of a particular disease. Regimen A requires prolonged hospitalization and leads to intractable vomiting, severe mouth ulcers, hair loss, and risk of life-threatening infection. Regimen B is administered on an outpatient basis, usually without serious toxicity. The choice is, as my residents would say, a "no-brainer." Another "no-brainer" is the choice between regimens of equal toxicity, when one regimen clearly has superior control or cure rates. The real world is often somewhere in between, and the particular choices made reflect the particular circumstances of a particular person at a particular time. (One of my patients was a concert violinist. The regimen she chose for the treatment of Hodgkin's Disease was more toxic than the alternative in most respects, but avoided the risk that accompanied the other regimen of damage to the nerves in her fingers.) In quality of life considerations, it is in the trade-off between morbidity and mortality, and in the comparison of people rather than treatments, that most of the ethical dilemmas arise.

It should be noted that the phrase "sanctity of life" is not without its own problems. Hauerwas offers the following criticism:

> The phrase "sanctity of life," when separated from its theological context, became an ideological slogan for a narrow individualism antithetical to the Christian way of life. Put starkly, Christians are not fundamentally concerned about living. Rather, their concern is to die for the right thing. Appeals to the sanctity of life as an ideology make it appear that Christians are committed to the proposition that there is nothing in life worth dying for.[14]

Keyserlingk says:

> The Christian view is somewhat ambivalent about death. On the one hand death is seen as a punishment for original sin and not at all natural.
>
> But on the other hand, Christians believe in salvation and immortality which should endow death with a dignity and even a certain attraction. Yet as one theologian writes, "How striking it is that those who profess faith in personal survival after biological death are often the ones who hang on most grimly and desperately to biological life in spite of the end of personal integrity."[15]

C. S. Lewis provides an interesting perspective:

> Ordinary men have not been so much in love with life as is usually supposed: small as their share of it is, they have found it too much to bear without reducing a large portion of it as nearly to non-life as they can: we love drugs, sleep, irresponsibility, amusement, are more than half in love with easeful death—if only we could be sure it wouldn't hurt! Only He who [fully] lived a human life (and I presume that only one did) can fully taste the horror of death.[16]

In an article entitled "Second Thoughts About Body Parts," Gilbert Meilaender warns that, in transplant medicine, our society presses toward a vision of humanity in which everyone becomes "a useful precadaver." . . . The truth is, we will do almost anything to keep ourselves or our loved ones alive. Whatever we may think public policy ought to be, if our own life or our child's were at stake, we might well bend our entire energies to the task of finding an organ for transplant. Whatever could be done we would be tempted to do, and we are therefore helpless in the face of the relentless advance of this technology. Christians, who know that death is indeed an evil and the last enemy opposed to God's will for the creation, should find the temptation quite understandable.

But we also need to develop the trust and the courage that will enable us sometimes to decline to do what medical technology makes possible. There are circumstances in which we can save life—even our own or that of a loved one—only by destroying the kind of world in which we all should want to live. In learning to say no, in becoming people who give thanks for medical progress but do not worship it or place our trust in it, we may bear a different kind of life-giving witness to the world.[17]

Hauerwas agrees "that while we do not wish to die, we do not oppose death as if life were an end in itself."[18]

So, I uphold the principle of the sanctity of life when it is firmly tethered to its Scriptural roots. I submit that the concept of quality of life—properly construed—need not violate it. Is any of this important in the real world? Let me tell you about Lisa.

Lisa[19] was in her early twenties when I first met her. She and Dan had just celebrated their first anniversary. She was eleven weeks pregnant, having had a miscarriage a few months earlier. Routine prenatal lab tests had suggested an abnormality of her blood cells, so I was asked to see her. A bone marrow test confirmed what she least wanted to hear: she had acute myeloid leukaemia. Without treatment, she would die within weeks. Standard treatment offered a long-term survival rate of about 25%. It would entail at least three cycles of intense multi-drug chemotherapy, given four to six weeks apart, and consideration of bone marrow transplantation.

Following an intense review of the literature and much discussion, it was agreed that we would delay for one week, until Lisa was past twelve weeks gestation, and then proceed with the first course of standard chemotherapy. My concern for her was heightened by the fact that the particular sub-type of leukaemia she had was particularly prone to cause severe bleeding problems.

Lisa's first cycle of treatment and recovery was relatively uneventful, even boring. She and Dan spent hours playing backgammon and dominoes. (They even taught me how to play!) She was discharged from hospital in less than four weeks in complete remission. That was the good news. A few days later, the obstetrician called to say that Lisa had had a miscarriage the night before. No specific cause was identified.

We proceeded with the second cycle of chemotherapy. It was a little more toxic than the first, but not enough to interfere with some serious domino tournaments. (I was starting to get the hang of it. She even let me win now and then!) Lisa was soon back on her feet physically and emotionally. Her equanimity was remarkable. In addition to the usual toxicities, the third cycle of chemotherapy was followed by an episode of bleeding into her lungs and a brief period of ventilator support. Again, once the toxicities subsided, Lisa recovered quickly.

Shortly thereafter, Lisa and Dan drove out to the transplant centre for a consultation concerning the role of a bone marrow transplant for Lisa, either immediately or in the event of a relapse. While she was there, she was found to have evidence of recurrent hepatitis, presumably transfusion-associated, what we now call hepatitis C. This would have made a transplant particularly risky, so she was sent to see a liver specialist who advised that she begin a three month course of Interferon treatments immediately. The specialist was quite miffed when Lisa insisted on discussing his advice with me by telephone from his office before she would agree to follow it.

When I saw Lisa a few weeks later, she had some flu-like symptoms, which is not unusual while taking Interferon. She had more nausea than is usual, though, and the explanation was unexpected: She was pregnant again. (I teased her that they should have stuck to dominoes!) There was almost no information available about the effects of Interferon in pregnancy. Lisa's liver inflammation had settled, so we stopped the Interferon, told the transplant centre to take her off their list for the time being, and waited. Lisa was twenty-two weeks pregnant when her leukaemia relapsed.

On the advice of the obstetrician and the neonatologist, we agreed to try supportive care alone until twenty-eight weeks, but the bleeding complications that accompanied the disease became uncontrollable by week twenty-three, so chemotherapy was started. At week twenty-four, infected and bleeding, Lisa went into premature labour and the baby died *in utero*. When Lisa was well enough to attend, a funeral service was held in the hospital chapel. A couple of weeks later, she was on her way back to the transplant centre.

Lisa weathered the bone marrow transplant and returned home. The next sixteen months were a fairly quiet, medically: a little hepatitis, some septic arthritis, and antibiotic allergies; troublesome but manageable. Lisa and Dan packed a lot of living into that time. When Lisa's leukaemia relapsed a second time, there was a new drug available that she hadn't yet received. Although she understood that a cure was no longer a possibility—that we would only be buying time—she said, "Let's go for it." This round was much more difficult than previous cycles, including a prolonged stay in the Intensive Care Unit and many days of ventilator support. One day, while she was on the ventilator, I asked, "So how are you doing, really?" Unable to speak, she wrote, "Know Monty Python?" I admitted that I did. She replied, "Not dead yet!" I got the message.

When Lisa had recovered enough to read a newspaper, she was dismayed to find that Garth Brooks was coming to town for a concert three months later, and that Dan had missed the opportunity to get tickets. As we discussed discharge plans, she gave us our orders: Dan was to get his hands on some tickets, and I was to make sure she lived long enough to get to the concert. We both did as we were told, and I heard all the happy details at her monthly visit to the clinic. Three weeks after the concert, Lisa's leukaemia relapsed yet again and she died quietly a few days later.

Maybe I should have called this discussion, "Lessons Learned from Lisa." The first lesson was that the right thing to do is to do the right thing. My local colleagues in clinical haematology were unanimous in their opinion that Lisa should have a surgical abortion before she received any chemotherapy. Medical intuition suggested that drugs designed to interfere with rapid cell growth were not to be given to a pregnant woman. The literature told a different story: that the drugs Lisa needed had been used in pregnancy, and that the babies had either been born healthy or not at all. A surgical abortion in the setting of low blood counts and impaired blood clotting would have been associated with a very high risk of bleeding and infection. The spontaneous abortion occurred at a time when Lisa's blood was fully normal. It was tragic, but it was safe. My colleagues thought the outcome was the same. Lisa knew better. She knew that she had given her child a chance, and her grieving wasn't complicated by guilt.

Lisa did a better job than many of really living while she was dying. At every point, she made life-affirming choices. She was also a realist, who met the tough issues head-on, made the best decisions she could, and never looked back. Her vocabulary didn't include the phrase "if only." Her Christian faith was uncomplicated and rock-solid. When she read in Siegel's book *Love, Medicine and Miracles* about his inner guide named George,[20] she tossed the book into the garbage, saying, "The only inner guide I'm going to listen to doesn't go by the name of George!"

Most of Lisa's adult, married life was an enormous struggle. You may be wondering if she thought it was worth it. It was a question we never discussed directly, although I believe her answer was clear in the choices she made. She expressed her opinion when she planned her funeral. It was, for the most part, a traditional requiem for the dead. It ended, though, with a Garth Brooks song. Recall, as you consider the lyrics, that Lisa knew "chance" by a more certain Name:

> Looking back on the memory of
>> the dance we shared with all the stars above.
> For a moment, all the world was right.
> How could I have known that you'd ever say goodbye?
>> And now, I'm glad I didn't know
>>> the way it all would end, the way it all would go.
>> Our lives are better left to chance.
> I could have missed the pain,
>> but I'd have had to miss the dance.
> Holding you, I held everything.

For a moment, wasn't I the king?

If I'd only known how the king would fall.

Hey, who's to say? You know I might have changed it all.[21]

Being Lisa's physician was one of the most difficult and most rewarding tasks of my professional life. David Stevens, the executive director of CMDS-US, says that Christian physicians should be set apart from our colleagues by certain distinguishing marks: excellence, humility, compassion, transparency, and charity.[22] Because I'm the story-teller here, I don't have to tell you the stories in which I got it mostly wrong. With Lisa, by the grace of God, I think I got it mostly right.

Caring for Lisa demanded more than simple competence. She pushed me to pursue excellence in the practice of clinical haematology. However, Lisa needed expertise well beyond my own, and there was no room for arrogance on the part of her attending physician. It was relatively easy to be transparent with Lisa, because of her own transparency. What she needed most from me, though, was compassion and love. She needed me to be there with her for the long haul, especially when there was nothing I could do. The pain, the suffering, the grief, the losses that she experienced were sometimes almost more than I could bear. It was tempting to retreat. It was tempting to give up. It was tempting to give in to the attitude around us that saw her struggle from a safe distance, and questioned if it was worth it. The church (with a small "c") was essential to my well-being during my years as Lisa's physician. Throughout that time, my cell group sustained me with their love and their presence and their prayers. And God was faithful to fill my emptiness and inadequacy with his all-sufficient love for Lisa.

Perhaps if I had read Hauerwas before I met Lisa, I'd have been better prepared. Or, perhaps Lisa prepared me to hear what Hauerwas has to say:

> The physician's basic pledge is not to cure, but to care through being present to the one in pain. Yet it is not easy to carry out that commitment on a day-to-day basis. For none of us has the resources to see too much pain without that pain hardening us. Without such a hardening, something we sometimes call by the name of professional distance, we fear we will lose the ability to

feel at all. . . .

Medicine is first of all pledged to be nothing more than a human presence in the face of suffering. . . . To learn how to be present in that way we need examples— that is, a people who have so learned to embody such a presence in their lives that it has become the marrow of their habits. The church at least claims to be such a community, as it is a group of people called out by a God who, we believe, is always present to us, both in our sin and our faithfulness. Because of God's faithfulness we are supposed to be a people who have learned how to be faithful to one another by our willingness to be present, with all our vulnerabilities, to one another. For what does our God require of us other than our unfailing presence in the midst of the world's sin and pain? Thus our willingness to be ill and to ask for help, as well as our willingness to be present with the ill is no special or extraordinary activity, but a form of the Christian obligation to be present to one another in and out of pain. . . .

Thus medicine needs the church . . . as a resource of the habits and practices necessary to sustain the care of those in pain over the long haul. For it is no easy matter to be with the ill, especially when we cannot do much for them other than simply be present. Our very helplessness too often turns to hate, both toward the one in pain and ourselves, as we despise them for reminding us of our helplessness. Only when we remember that our presence is our doing, when sitting on the ground seven days saying nothing is what we can do, can we be saved from our fevered and hopeless attempt to control others' and our own existence. Of course to believe that such presence is what we can and should do entails a belief in a presence in and beyond this world. And it is certainly true many today no longer believe in or experience such a presence. If that is the case, then I do wonder if medicine as an activity of presence is possible in a world without God.[23]

This kind of involvement with patients is contrary to much of the advice I received when I began my training. I was delighted when I discovered Diane Komp's books, because in them I find permission to ignore such advice. Dr. Komp is a children's cancer specialist. She writes:

> To be exposed to suffering children is a dangerous proposition. As children died, my faith seemed to . . . perish as well. To handle the pain, I took the advice of a professor of internal medicine.
>
> He was doing his best to counsel young students. . . . He advised us not to heed the pain that our feelings bring when we listen to our patients. We should simply do our work and concentrate on that. Hard work is a good tonic for untamed and uneasy feelings. There was plenty of work, ample opportunity to concentrate away from the untidy area of emotion . . .
>
> I learned to work unflogged by untidy feelings. But every time I considered taking a "safe" course, to avoid the suffering of children, the path led away from the most joyous parts of medicine as well. . . .
>
> I think back on the pain that I tried to avoid by distancing myself from these children and realize how much greater the pain of avoidance is than that of their embrace. . . . Young doctors with other options count themselves privileged to cast their lot with these children. And middle-aged physicians like me can find our way back to faith when we listen to such children.
>
> Therein is the paradox: The closer you come . . . the less the pain. If you risk letting your heart be broken, you just may find it healed.[24]

How, then, should we live? What is our task as Christian physicians? How do we uphold the sanctity of life and enhance quality of life in a culture of death? I think David Stevens is right. I think our task is to pursue professional excellence, to be Christ-like in our humility, to risk the vulnerability of genuine compassion and transparency, and to give sacrificially all that we have and all that we are. The CMDS logo is a cross, a basin, and a towel. Jesus is our role model for this task of sacrificial love and humble service. But I admit that there are days when this task is overwhelming. For those days—and I'll end with this—let me suggest that you learn to play dominoes:

> For the beauty of dominoes is that any one can play the game. You have but to grasp two essential principles. You must clearly understand in the first place that, at every turn, you must match your companion's play, lay-ing a six beside his six, a three beside his three, and so on. And you must clearly understand in the second place that the whole secret of success lies, not in hoard-ing, but in spending. Victory lies in paying out the little ivory tablets with as prodigal a hand as possible. It is better in dominoes to give than to keep. It is better to play a domino with twelve black dots on it than a dom-ino with only two. . . . Life itself is but a game of domi-noes. Its highest art lies in matching your companion's pieces. Is he glad? It is a great thing to be able to rejoice with those who do rejoice. Is he sad? It is a great thing to be able to weep with those that weep. It means, of course, that if you answer the challenge every time, your pieces will soon be gone. But . . . it is worth remember-ing that victory lies not in accumulation, but in exhaus-tion. The player who is first left with empty hands wins everything.[25]

Notes

[1] J. Christodoulou et al., "Early Treatment of Classical Menkes Disease with Par-enteral Copper-Histidine: Some Benefits, but Substantial Persisting Abnor-malities" (unpublished draft).

[2] R. Massie and S. Massie, *Journey* (New York: Alfred A. Knopf, 1975), 244-45.

[3] E. W. Keyserlingk, *Sanctity of Life or Quality of Life in the Context of Ethics, Medi-cine and Law* (Ottawa: Law Reform Commission of Canada, 1975), 11.

[4] P. Ramsey, "The Morality of Abortion," in *Moral Problems: A Collection of Philo-sophical Essays*, ed. J. Rachels (New York: Harper & Row, 1971), 11-12.

[5] K. Barth, *Church Dogmatics*, vol. 3, part 4, (Edinburgh: T&T Clark, 1961), 339.

[6] N. St. John-Stevas, *The Right to Life* (New York: Holt, Rinehart and Winston, 1964), 12.

[7] Ramsey, 13.

8 Keyserlingk, 13.

9 Ibid., 50.

10 Editorial, *California Medicine*, (September 1970), 67–68.

11 Keyserlingk, 51–52.

12 Ibid., 53.

13 Ibid., 59–60.

14 S. Hauerwas, *Suffering Presence* (Notre Dame, Ind.: University of Notre Dame Press, 1986), 92.

15 Keyserlingk, 67.

16 C. S. Lewis, *A Mind Awake* (New York.: Harcourt Brace Jovanovich, Harvest Edition, 1980), 99.

17 G. Meilaender, "Second Thoughts About Body Parts," *First Things* 62 (1996): 37.

18 Hauerwas, 98.

19 Names and minor details have been changed.

20 B. S. Siegel, *Love, Medicine and Miracles* (New York: Harper & Row, 1986), 20.

21 "The Dance," words and music by Tony Arata, ©1989 Morganactive Songs, Inc./Pookie Bear Music (ASCAP). All rights reserved. Used by permission. Warner Bros. Publications US Inc., Miami, Fla. 33014.

22 D. Stevens, "What Is the King Going to Say?" *Physician* 8, no. 3 (1996): 9–10.

23 Hauerwas, 79–81.

24 D. M. Komp, *A Child Shall Lead Them: Lessons in Hope from Children with Cancer* (Grand Rapids, Mich.: Zondervan, 1993), 37, 42, 43. See also D. M. Komp, *A Window to Heaven: When Children See Life in Death* (Grand Rapids, Mich.: Zondervan, 1992).

25 F. W. Boreham, *The Silver Shadow and Other Day Dreams* (New York: Abingdon Press, 1918), 12, 16.

Howie Bright

Natural Family Planning

Christians are taking a second look at contraception. The past generation has viewed contraception as acceptable, and some churches have even promoted its use as responsible behaviour. But now many people blame a contraceptive mentality, and the irresponsible behaviour it encourages, for the moral decline so widely evident in our day. Christian physicians are increasingly aware of abortifacient effects of contraceptives, as well as deleterious effects on the health of women. There is certainly a need for responsible family planning, but can this be done in a way that avoids the physical harms and moral harms of contraception? Natural family planning has provided the answer: it allows *more effective* family planning than is available from any artificial method, and it allows complete harmony with God's plan for marriage.

This paper will review (briefly) the most popular method of natural family planning (NFP), and will present the scientific evidence which verifies its efficacy. We will also consider the moral issues involved with contraception, and demonstrate that NFP encourages a fully Christian married life.

What is Natural Family Planning?

NFP has been defined as planning to achieve or avoid pregnancy by the timing of intercourse according to the fertile phase of the menstrual cycle.[1] Infertile couples can use the method to achieve pregnancy, and couples desiring to postpone childbearing can use the same method for this purpose. We tend to think of NFP in terms of pregnancy avoidance, but really it's a method of *fertility recognition* that can be used either way. Most of this discussion will be about the use of NFP for pregnancy avoidance, but I'd like to emphasize at the outset that it works both ways.[2]

Women are fertile for a brief time during each cycle, because the ovum survives for less than twenty-four hours after ovulation, and maximal sperm survival is five days. There are reliable natural indicators which allow women to recognize their fertile time. Couples can choose to abstain from intercourse during this time if they wish to avoid pregnancy: this is NFP in a nutshell! So what are these natural indicators, and how reliable are they?

The oldest method of periodic abstinence is calendar rhythm, where women expect ovulation at mid-cycle and use a calendar to estimate their fertile time. This method has a 20% pregnancy rate, because the timing of ovulation is variable. The Planned Parenthood Federation persists, even in their 1996 literature, in calling NFP "the rhythm method." This is wrong and represents either unconscionable ignorance or wilful deceit on the part of Planned Parenthood, an important promoter of the contraceptive industry.[3] *NFP is not the rhythm method!*

The post-ovulatory rise in basal body temperature has been recognized for a century. R. Röetzer was the first to apply this knowledge to family planning.[4] From his work have evolved various natural methods which rely on the thermal shift, such as the sympto-thermal method, or the Serena Method in Canada. There is still no consensus on the best way to determine pre- and postovulatory phases by means of the thermal shift, although the variations of this method have been extensively researched.[5] The problems relating to this method are that the Basal Body Temperature (BBT) rise is imprecisely related in timing to the LH surge which triggers ovulation: the thermal shift can occur as early as three days before to three days after the LH peak.[6] Also, BBT as a marker is subject to extraneous influences, such as drugs, viremia, or activity. Another problem with temperature methods occurs when cycles become prolonged, such as in the perimenopausal years or during lactation.[7] Despite these difficulties, however, the method is widely and successfully used, especially in Europe.

John Billings, an Australian neurologist, pioneered the use of cervical mucus observations to predict ovulation, and thereby to allow natural family planning.[8] Mucus is continually produced in crypts which line the cervical canal. Chemically, mucus is a gel, consisting of solid and liquid phases. The solid phase is a glycoprotein polymer called mucin. The liquid phase has water-soluble proteins, enzymes, and salts. The production and composition of mucus is under hormonal control. Whenever total oestrogens exceed a threshold of 15 mg/100 ml/day, the cervical mucus is sufficiently liquefied to leave the cervix and appear at the vulva. If a cycle is ovulatory, the mucus becomes increasingly lubricative and stretchy and clear until it reaches its "peak." The peak is defined as the last day of lubricative mucus, and this signal corresponds with remarkable precision to the LH surge. Ovulation follows the LH surge by sixteen hours.

In this method, women are taught to observe their mucus symptoms at the vulva, especially sensations of wetness and lubricativeness, or of dryness. Visual observation of the mucus after a wipe with toilet paper, and feeling with fingertip will confirm *spinnbarkeit*. When clear, stretchy, lubricative mucus is present at the vulva, women are fertile. For most of the month, mucus is thick, opaque, and non-stretchy. This infertile mucus acts as an impenetrable barrier to sperm, causing them to be destroyed by the acid vaginal pH within an hour or two. When fertile mucus appears, however, sperm survival and motility are greatly enhanced. While it was John who had the original insight into the usefulness of these observations for family planning, it was really his wife, Dr. Lyn Billings, who developed an effective way to teach women about this method.[9] Charts are used with different stickers for menses, dryness, fertile mucus, and infertile mucus; this provides a record which allows accurate determination of fertility or infertility at any time of the month.

Our knowledge about structure and properties of cervical mucus is based on the work of Dr. Eric Odeblad, a Lutheran gynaecologist from Sweden. Since there is precious little clinical work available for a pro-life gynaecologist in Sweden, Odeblad has devoted his entire career to research on cervical mucus. He has identified several types of mucus, produced in separate crypts, which vary cyclically. The most important of these are G, L, and S mucus, which have different ions bound to their proteins and varying water content. G mucus is formed under progesterone influence from lower crypts; the particle structure is like a dense mesh which acts as a barrier. S mucus is formed under oestrogen stimulation; it has high water content and low viscosity, with particles aligned into linear channels which facilitate sperm transport. L mucus is also triggered by oestrogen, and appears microscopically as bead-like structures on the strands of S mucus; these beads actually select out imperfect sperm forms. The relative amounts of G, S, and L mucus at any time determine a woman's fertility.[10]

Dr. James Brown is a research endocrinologist who has worked with the Billings at Melbourne. He performed hormone assays on thousands of women who charted their mucus symptoms, and proved the close connection between the LH surge, ovulation, and observation of the peak mucus signal. His work was first published in *Lancet* in 1972.[11] This connection has been proven in many subsequent studies, including work by Hilgers[12] who used ultrasound observations of ovulation to confirm the precision of mucus signs in identifying ovulation.

Women can easily be taught to recognize their mucus symptoms. Because fertile mucus *predicts* ovulation, it can be used for women whose cycles are irregular, or where ovulation is delayed by lactation, discontinuing oral contraceptives, and in the perimenopausal years. The method is successfully used by blind women, and millions of illiterate women in third world countries. If they wish to avoid pregnancy, they must abstain from intercourse, from the first day of fertile mucus until the fourth day after the peak. Five or six days is the average time that women observe fertile mucus, although for some women it may only appear for a few hours each month, or every several months for the relatively infertile. Because abstinence is involved, the method requires communication and loving co-operation from the husband. Some detractors of the method[13] claim that men cannot co-operate in this way, but proponents see this requirement for co-operation as a strength of NFP:

> Understanding and co-operation are necessary for natural family planning to work, but also for relationships to work. Couples in which women are forced to submit to men for sex require counselling, not pills, which only perpetuate destructive attitudes likely to result in further misery and break-down of trust. Sexual intercourse is supposed to be an intimate expression of love, a choice freely made, and not a means of using others to satisfy an "irresistible" physiological urge.[14]

Worldwide, a 1993 survey suggests that 49% of women aged fifteen to forty-nine use some form of reversible contraception, and 14% rely on some method of periodic abstinence for family planning.[15] In North America, these figures are 59.2% and 2.7% respectively. NFP is cheaper, safer, and more effective than contraception but there is clearly a long way to go in promoting it. There is a bias against natural methods, there is fear of abstinence, and there has been an unwarranted delay in gaining acceptance into medical curricula, but things are starting to change. The 1990 multinational conference on NFP which took place at Georgetown University[16] and recent positive reviews in the *BMJ*[17] and *Lancet*[18] show that the simple facts of fertility awareness are at last gaining recognition in the scientific community.

Scientific Trials

Let's look at published evidence on NFP. We must first acknowledge a large caveat: the assumption that couples studied wish to avoid pregnancy. If a couple enrols in an NFP study, their initial intention may well be to avoid pregnancy. But they have an option at any time to change their mind; the NFP couple is always open to new life. It seems improper to call pregnancy a "failure" when this could well have been the couple's deliberate choice at that moment. However, this is the language employed by researchers into efficacy of family planning methods, so we must accept this grain of salt as we study the literature.

There are two statistics considered in all trials, whether NFP or contraception: total pregnancy rate and method pregnancy rate (MPR). The MPR refers to pregnancies that occur despite perfect use of a method. Pregnancies occur with any method, even sterilization, for reasons that are unknown. MPR's widely publicized for oral contraceptives are based on old trials of high dose pills; it is surprisingly hard to find studies of the newer low dose triphasic pills, and most authorities still publish MPR of 0.5 for BCP. This compares to MPR in published ovulation method trials of 0 to 2.7.[19]

The other important statistic is the total pregnancy rate, usually expressed as the Pearl Index (PI). This includes all "failures," whether the method is used properly or improperly, for one hundred women using the method over one year. Most pregnancies in any method occur early in the use of the method, when couples are inexperienced. The longer a method is used, the lower the PI becomes. It is worth considering, when reviewing any published trial, whether couples enrolled into the study are experienced users (as with most BCP trials) or new users of the method.

A recent literature search showed twenty-six published trials of NFP, but the most famous is the World Health Organization (WHO) trial, which started in 1976. This was a prospective trial for two years involving nine hundred women from five countries (India, New Zealand, Ireland, El Salvador, and the Philippines). To be enrolled in the study women had to be of proven fertility, have cycles lasting twenty-three to thirty-five days, and they must have had no prior knowledge of the method. The reason for this last inclusion criterion was that the investigators wanted to study how readily the method could be learned. Their conclusions were that the method was indeed easy to learn, with 93% correctly charting their mucus signs after a single teaching session. The method pregnancy rate was a reasonable 2.4%, but the PI was high at 20%.[20]

This high PI from the WHO study engendered a general bias in the scientific community that NFP was impractical because of an unacceptably high pregnancy rate. As was noted earlier, this bias is changing slowly as a result of more recent, and better, trials and the work of Dr. James Trussell, a statistician from Princeton. He went back to the WHO study and looked at the data more critically.[21] His concerns were that there was no control for lactation (and mucus signs may be harder to interpret during lactation); it's unfair to publish a PI for inexperienced users of a method; and he questioned the validity of the couple's stated intention to avoid pregnancy at the outset (ambivalent couples may be more prone to risk-taking). After a critical re-examination of the data, Trussell noted that 87% of the cycles were characterized by perfect use of the method, with a PI <2%, but 13% of the cycles were characterized by imperfect use. Breaking the peak rule carries a 27% risk of pregnancy (67% on the peak day itself!) and this had a large impact on the overall failure rate observed in the study. He concluded that the "ovulation method is quite effective at preventing pregnancy when used properly, but is extremely unforgiving of imperfect use."[22]

Trussell's conclusions are borne out by all of the recent published trials. The largest of these was from India involving twenty thousand impoverished and illiterate women in Calcutta, who achieved a total pregnancy rate of only 0.2%![23] The success here is attributed to high motivation from poverty, and excellent support from well-trained NFP teachers. There was an interesting study in Italy[24] where couples enrolled were asked whether their motivation was to space out their childbearing, or to avoid any further pregnancies. The total pregnancy rate for the first group was 3.6 but in the second group was 0! These and other recent trials show that NFP is *at least* as effective as any artificial method of contraception. We have a lot of scientific ammunition in discussing NFP with our patients.

Another statistic should be considered with reference to methods of family planning: continuation rate. With Norplant[25] the one year continuation rate is 50%, and is 70% for BCP (to age thirty-five only). Most NFP trials have shown much higher continuation rates. The first couples in the Melbourne centre showed a 98% *four year* continuation rate.[26] I believe that this high level of user satisfaction derives not so much from confidence in the efficacy of NFP—though this confidence is justified by the published trials. Rather it derives from an enhanced marital relationship fostered by the use of this method.

Moral Considerations

Sex is God's great gift to mankind. He allows man to share in his creative power, and it is clearly his wish that we do so, for he commands us to "Be fruitful and multiply, and fill the earth and subdue it" (Gen 1:28).[27] God is present in the conjugal act between husband and wife, as Eve recognizes in her joyful cry on the occasion of the very first human birth: "I have produced a man with the help of the Lord" (Gen 4:1). Not every conjugal act results in conception, but spouses should acknowledge God's creative power in their sexual relations, and they should not be deliberately thwarting this power. Those acts of intercourse which do not result in conception, but which remain open to the possibility of new life, will powerfully express the love of husband and wife for each other. This is also part of God's plan: the sexual act is a physical expression of human love, and it strengthens spouses in their love. "Therefore a man leaves his father and his mother and clings to his wife, and they become one flesh" (Gen 2:24).

Thus the traditional view of sexual intercourse describes both its unitive and procreative aspects. This is how sex was designed by God for mankind. But Adam and Eve wanted to be gods unto themselves, and brought about the fall of mankind through their original sin. So it is that contraception thwarts God's design for sex; there is a desire to have the unitive benefit of sex without the procreative. But you can't have one without the other, as we are finding out to our cost nowadays. When we destroy God's plan for sex we lose even the unitive benefit of conjugal relations. Sex becomes cheap, a mere release of an urge, not a mutual total gift of self, deepening the love of spouses for each other. Contracepted sex is a mere pantomime of real sex.

> In coition the woman gives and surrenders herself to the man by complete openness, receptiveness, submission, and a full unfolding of herself to this sole partner. The man, on his part, gives himself to the woman through his entrancement with her, his finding satisfaction in her alone, his yearning to protect her, his permeation and penetration of her with his very substance, his focussing all his attention and activity exclusively upon this one woman. Moreover, coitus is the physiological act of procreation. The yielding of one's body is the natural symbol of willingness to become father or mother, of yearning to make one's partner father or mother, of the love that desires that exalted physical, mental, and spiritual maturity for one's partner which comes only from parenthood. Coition is not merely the condition for but the symbol of the creative act of God. Coition is *procreation*; God alone creates.[28]

A biblical description of spousal love so ordered is given in the account of the wedding night of Tobiah (Tob 8:4-9). Contrast this beautiful description of married love with contracepted intercourse:

> The woman who uses a diaphragm has closed herself to her husband. She has accepted his affection but not his substance. The same is true for a man who uses a condom. He worships her with his body but not enough to share with her his substance. He takes no responsibility

for her. Thus, such mates perform what appears to be an act of love but is only a sham; they lie to one another in their bodies as in their hearts. They take that which says perfect union and corrupt it till it can express only mutual pleasure.[29]

Some have argued that man should be allowed to regulate birth by artificial means, since God, after all, gave man dominion over nature in the Old Testament. But there are limits to our active intervention. Artificial birth control represents similar sinfulness as suicide or euthanasia in which we act as if we are the masters of life. Contraception is "no mere biological intervention but the severing of a bond which is under the jurisdiction of God alone."[30] "So they are no longer two but one flesh. What therefore God has joined together, let no man put asunder" (Mk 10:8-9 RSV).

The story of Onan (Gen 38:8-10) shows that God's people from the earliest days regarded contraception as a sin. Contraception was universally opposed by Protestant churches until the Anglican conference at Lambeth in 1930, when contraception in marriage was permitted in certain limited circumstances—the thin edge of the wedge.[31] A 1989 book[32] lists ninety-nine Protestant theologians who taught against onanism. Luther, Calvin, and Wesley were strongly opposed to unnatural birth control, with Luther calling it a form of sodomy, Calvin calling it the murder of future persons, and Wesley saying it could destroy your soul. There was not a single Protestant theologian who defended contraception prior to the 1930s.

This all changed with the advent of oral contraceptives in the 1960s. It *appeared* that there was openness between spouses and God during conjugal relations. In February 1961 the General Council of Churches endorsed the use of artificial contraception as part of responsibility in family planning.[33] There was widespread expectation that the Catholic Church would also fall into line with this trend. Despite pressure from the world and from within its own ranks, the Church reaffirmed her traditional teaching regarding contraception with the encyclical *Humanae vitae*, released by Pope Paul VI on July 25, 1968. The Church's stand was clarified and expressed powerfully in this document. Of course, all that mattered was the bottom line, that contraception was still proscribed for Catholics, and very few people actually read the encyclical.

Most people believed sincerely that oral contraceptives would strengthen marriage through liberation from the threat of childbearing. Pope Paul predicted in *Humanae vitae* that precisely the opposite would occur:

> Indeed, it is to be feared that husbands who become accustomed to contraceptive practices will lose respect for their wives. They may come to disregard their wife's psychological and physical equilibrium and use their wives as instruments for serving their own desires. Consequently, they will no longer view their wives as companions who should be treated with attentiveness and love.[34]

At the time Pope Paul made this prophecy, he was universally derided and scorned. People everywhere, including many outspoken Catholics, genuinely believed that oral contraception was an important medical achievement that would foster harmony in marital relations. The Catholic Church was seen to be stuck in the dark ages, completely out of touch with modern realities. (As an aside, it's a pet peeve of mine how the media blame Catholics for breeding like rabbits at the same time as they poke fun at Catholics for universally ignoring the Church's ban on contraception!)

We all know too many abandoned women and broken homes. Infidelity is made easy by contraception. Divorce rates now approach 50% in Canada. Premarital sex is practically a norm. I don't need to remind a Christian audience about the indices of moral decay we all see every day. I think we have to acknowledge that Pope Paul's prophecy was all too correct, and that a contraceptive mentality is at least partly to blame for our present situation.

One can gain insight into the wrongness of contraception through philosophical reflection on the unitive and procreative meanings of sexual intercourse, but sometimes one can *just know* that it's wrong. I would cite the poignant stories of Ruth Lassiter[35] and Ellen Homan.[36] These women could sense their marriages were in trouble. Their husbands were faithful but sex was perfunctory; something was missing. Ultimately they knew they had to stop contracepting, and when they stated this to their husbands, both of these men realized they had been treating their women as sex objects for their own gratification.

Under the guise of helping love, artificial contraception cunningly establishes a tyrant in the marriage: the sex act declines from a reaffirming of the whole marriage covenant, true love-making, to joint seeking of mutual satisfaction. A subtle shift, but a decisive one, away from God and the covenant of marriage. The nuptial exchange between man and woman is replaced by a woman's sense, vague and miniscule at first, that she must be "available" to her husband; anxiety develops about "performance" and sensual attractiveness; she may begin to feel used by her spouse. The husband, in an equally subtle way, ceases to delight in his bride and begins to think of her as an object to arouse and satisfy his passion. He has a vague sense that something is wrong; he feels restless and unsatisfied.[37]

Stopping contraception enriched these marriages. There are many other such testimonies from couples who discover NFP. In fact, my wife's search for truth in these matters led me to finally read *Humanae vitae* and stop prescribing artificial contraception in my family practice. Doctors as well as husbands can be happier without contraception!

Once my wife and I were discussing this notion with a marriage preparation class at our church. Afterwards a young man berated me for insulting his parents, one of whom had been sterilized early in their marriage, but who enjoyed a long and happy life together. While I would not defend their action, I certainly don't wish to insult people who contracept or have themselves sterilized. I have patients and friends with apparently successful marriages despite contraception. Nevertheless, there is a large risk here that sex can become selfish. There's a huge difference between saying "Let's have sex" and "Let's be open to having a baby." Viewing one's spouse as co-creator of new life adds mystery and depth to marital relations that takes them far beyond merely genital contact.

The greatest expression of a person's desire to give himself is to give the seed of himself. Giving one's seed is much more significant, and in particular is much more real, than giving one's heart. I am yours, I give you my seed; this is not poetry, it is love. It is conjugal love embodied in a unique and privileged physical action whereby intimacy is expressed—I give you what I give no one—and unity is achieved.[38]

Fertility is a natural part of ourselves, given to us by God as the means by which we can be co-creators with him. It is a gift. Yet the contraceptive mentality regards fertility as a threat, and modern medicine treats it as a disease, dispensing potent medications or even surgery to destroy fertility. I'm blessed with four generous partners who disagree with me, but who allow me to practise medicine in accord with my own beliefs. They will occasionally tease me about being weird, but I respond in kind by quietly whispering at their shoulder "Fertility is not a disease" whenever I hear them phoning a BCP prescription or booking a vasectomy. I admit that my practice is out of step with modern medicine in this regard but I believe the pendulum will swing away from blind acceptance of contraception in the future.

Many well-meaning people are alarmed by the "population explosion" and depletion of the earth's resources. No matter what its intrinsic effects, they view contraception as crucial to solving this problem. Although modern demography calls into question the alarmist Malthusian views on population,[39] there certainly are some areas in our world with too many people and too little food or productive work. Population control may well be necessary in some places.

Another prediction Pope Paul made in *Humanae vitae* was that contraception would afford governments a coercive tool to be used against their citizens without regard to moral considerations.[40] The enforced sterilization program in India, and currently the compulsory abortion policy in China are examples of this prophecy in action.[41] If population control is necessary, why not use a means which is both effective and humane? The largest NFP trials have been in India, among populations largely illiterate, and yet the efficacy rates have been astonishing. Government policy should promote NFP, to allow individual families to decide the population issue, rather than impose coercion which is a greater burden to people than their scarce resources. NFP provides both family planning and population control without the moral, monetary, or psychological expense of contraception.[42]

Can individuals be responsible about parenthood? What is meant by responsible parenthood anyway? The contraceptive view is expressed by Alan Guttemacher, a former director of the Planned Parenthood Federation:

> What does one mean by responsible sexual behaviour? It does not preclude premarital sexual activity, for premarital sex is not inherently evil. It may be eminently right and proper when practiced by the right couple under the right circumstances. Whenever sex relations take place in or out of marriage, they are patently immoral if the most effective birth control technique is not used, unless the child is mutually desired. The first line of defense against undesired pregnancy must be *contraception*. For physical and psychic reasons, abortion must be relegated to backup status for failed, or failure to use, effective contraception.[43]

This view can be contrasted with a Christian view of responsible parenthood: "Do everything for the glory of God" (1 Cor 10:31). Couples are called upon to be open to God's will about children, and not to regard babies as a threat. This does *not* mean they should conceive as many children as biologically possible. Parents must be able to feed and educate their children, and this obligation sets limits to childbearing. However, it doesn't mean that a child's college tuition must be in the bank before the child is even conceived! Only with prayer can parents discern God's will for them. Being responsible parents means being open and generous towards God's plan for them.

The Church recognizes that serious reasons exist to postpone childbearing, and rarely, to avoid childbearing altogether.[44] NFP allows this family planning to take place without any deliberate interference in the true meaning of sexual intercourse. God's design is being respected, not thwarted.

Of course, this requires abstinence from sex during the days of fertility each month. Abstinence is not easy. It can be irritating and frustrating, especially for couples who are accustomed to contracepted sex being available at all times. Modern man wants instant gratification and comfort, easy answers and quick fixes; any form of mortification is contrary to modern instincts.

Yet abstinence *is* possible, and even beneficial. We are not animals, governed by our passions and at the whim of our urges. We are human beings, capable of reason to control our actions. Like other forms of self-denial such as dieting or a savings program, abstinence has benefits. We learn self-control, which can help us through many difficulties. We also learn to communicate our love in ways other than sexually; we have to talk to each other—there's nothing else to do! The days of abstinence each month are like a courtship time, and each month there's a honeymoon to look forward to. Sex becomes special; romance returns to married life.

> Truly, discipline of this sort—from which conjugal chastity shines forth—cannot be an obstacle to love. Rather, discipline imbues love with a deeper human meaning. Although such control requires continuous effort, it also helps the spouses become strong in virtue and makes them rich with spiritual goods. And this virtue fosters the fruits of tranquility and peace in the home and helps in the solving of difficulties of other kinds. It aids the spouses in becoming more tender with each other and more attentive to each other. It assists them in dispelling that inordinate self-love that is the enemy of true love.[45]

Self-mastery leads not to repression but to freedom, the freedom to express not lust, but love.[46] It is significant to note that divorce rates among couples who have practised NFP for at least a year are 1% or less.[47]

The abortion issue has been responsible for a new awakening about the wrongness of contraception. Janet Smith and John Haas are examples of important Christian writers who became opposed to contraception because it directly fosters abortion. How can this be? Would not a more widespread availability of contraception reduce the need for abortions? This is certainly the teaching of Planned Parenthood and of public educators wanting to install condom machines and birth control clinics in schools. They are throwing gasoline on the flames of teenage sex.

Abortions result from unwanted pregnancies, and most unwanted pregnancies are the result of sexual relations outside of marriage, and most sexual relationships outside of marriage are facilitated by the availability of contraception.[48] Studies show that 80% of women having abortions are contraceptively experienced.[49]

> The resolve to prevent a child from coming to be is often sufficiently strong that one will eliminate the child whose conception is not prevented. Therefore, in countries that admitted contraception for general use, the increasing number of abortions compelled authorities to make them legal. It is important to remember that at the very core of the contraceptive mentality is fear of something which is perfectly natural—babies.[50]

"I have set before you life and death, the blessing and the curse. Choose life, so that you and your descendants may live" (Deut 30:19). In his moving testimony about contraception, Dr. John Haas finds that this fear of babies is the most compelling argument for him:

> Reasonable human acts are those directed toward ends perceived as goods. And three fundamental goods or ends can be found to be inherent within our sexuality: sensual pleasure, friendship, and the child. But which of these most adequately and fundamentally explains our sexual natures? Sexual pleasure does not ultimately explain our natures as male and female since it can be achieved to some degree even in isolation. Friendship is a great good of our sexual natures, but we know it does not ultimately explain the differentiation of sexes since even homosexuals seek this end, even though they are never able adequately to realize it. Ultimately what explains the differentiation of our natures as a male and female is the child toward which our sexuality is ordered. This is all that is meant by the traditional formula that the primary (not exclusive) end of marriage is the procreation and education of children. It seems to me that what is fundamentally wrong with contraception is that it invariably treats the procreative good, the child, as though it were an evil.[51]

The question is often asked, understandably, about the difference between NFP and contraception. Couples who use NFP to postpone childbearing, after all, are acting with the same intention as couples who contracept: they both wish to avoid pregnancy. But if NFP and contraception are the same, why not use NFP, the method which is safer and more effective? When contracepting couples are asked this question, they squirm. They know there's a difference, but it's hard to articulate. They doubt their own ability to handle abstinence. There's an inherent Western scepticism of things natural being effective; they'd sooner rely on technology.

It's not the *purpose* which makes the methods different; they are essentially different as *means*. Contraception may be used for a good purpose, that is, to limit the size of a family where this limitation is necessary. But having a good purpose does not make contraception good;[52] the end does not justify the means.

The real difference between NFP and contraception is whether or not the true meaning of sexual intercourse is being distorted. In NFP there is respect for one's fertility as part of one's being, and acts of intercourse preserve the integrity of the unitive and procreative meaning of sex. In contraception, fertility is a threat which is deliberately thwarted, and acts of intercourse deny the procreative meaning of sex. There is a difference between non-procreative acts and anti-procreative acts. Refraining from intercourse is not contraceptive intercourse since it is not intercourse at all.[53] A couple cannot be acting against the procreative good when they are convinced that the act of intercourse cannot in this instance be procreative. This use of NFP is based on the recognition that not all acts of marital intercourse are fertile and that in those that are not, the other goods of marriage may be pursued without prejudice to the good of procreation.[54]

Well-meaning people who endorse contraception have no logical argument against perversions:

> If you can turn intercourse into something other than the reproductive type of act (I don't mean of course that every act is reproductive any more than every acorn leads to an oak tree, but it's the reproductive type of act) then why, if you can change it, should it be restricted to the married? If sexual union can be deliberately and totally divorced from fertility, then we may wonder why sexual union has got to be married union.[55]

And if sex is really just an instrument towards self-gratification, then what is wrong with masturbation? Homosexual intercourse? Multiple partners? The contraceptive idea of sex affords no reasoned argument against these immoral acts. This by no means suggests that people who contracept will do all these things, but they will have no solid reason against these things.

> What miserable messes people keep on making, to their own and others' grief, by dishonourable sexual relationships! The Devil has scored a great propaganda victory: everywhere it's suggested that the troubles connected with sex are all to do with frustration, with abstinence, with society's cruel and conventional disapproval. As if, if we could only do away with these things, it would be a happy and life-enhancing romp for everyone; and as if all who were chaste were unhappy, not only unhappy but hard-hearted and censorious and nasty. The trouble with the Christian standard of chastity is that it isn't and never has been generally lived by; *not* that it would be profitless if it were. Quite the contrary: it would be colossally productive of earthly happiness.[56]

Those who have followed the footnotes to this paper will have noticed how heavily we have drawn from the work of Janet Smith, the University of Dallas professor of philosophy who has so staunchly and so eloquently explained the Church's teaching on contraception. We will conclude with an excerpt from one of her essays, which neatly summarizes our theme that NFP encourages a fully Christian married life:

> God is a silent partner in sex. God is the one who created male and female and made sexuality the most profound way in which their bodies communicate. He wrote into the sex act its meaning of union and procreation. Those practicing contraception are betraying and misusing a good which God has given to them. One of the goods they are denying is the good of parenthood. Children are a gift from God, not a punishment, as today's world so often thinks. Children are a gift which brings to true fruition the loving union of a couple. God has chosen to bring new life into the world through the union of lovers and to deny Him the op-

portunity to work in this fashion is to abuse the meaning which He has written into sex. Sex without contraception, then, carries with it the opportunity for the most profound expression of one's gift of oneself to another; one is not holding back one's own fertility—which is an integral part of oneself—nor is one refusing to accept the fertility of one's beloved partner. The couple does not tell God that they are dissatisfied with the way He arranged matters, but work in co-operation with the arrangement God has established.[57]

Further Reading

The best discussion of the ovulation method for patients is Lyn Billings' book, co-authored with Ann Westmore, *The Billings Method*. For medical readers wishing to learn the method, I strongly recommend the *Atlas of the Ovulation Method*, written by the doctors Billings and Maurice Catarinich. It contains sample charts representing normal and unusual menstrual cycles, and includes an appendix written by Eric Odeblad about the science of cervical mucus.

A concise summary of the scientific trials is presented in the paper by Ryder which appeared in the *BMJ* in 1993. An excellent survey of all the methods of NFP, extensively referenced, is Dr. Hanna Klaus' *Natural Family Planning: A Review*.

For the moral considerations, we relied heavily on the book edited by Janet Smith, *Why Humanae vitae Was Right*. Also useful is the Princeton symposium *Trust the Truth*, which took place in 1988 to commemorate the twentieth anniversary of *Humanae vitae*. All of these works are fully referenced in the endnotes which follow.

If the reader can find time to read just one reference from this paper, then let it be the encyclical *Humanae vitae* itself. Often people assume that papal encyclicals are dry and weighty tomes that are laborious to get through. In fact, *Humanae vitae* is beautifully written, and surprisingly brief. Re-reading it for this presentation, including note-taking, took only forty minutes. Section Nine of this document contains a description of human love which I feel can stand with the most beautiful expressions in all of literature.

Notes

1 Hanna Klaus, *Natural Family Planning: A Review*, 2nd ed. (Bethesda, Md.: NFP Center of Washington, D.C., 1995), 1.

2 In the United States, 10% of self-referrals to NFP clinics, and 90% of physician referrals, are for infertility (ibid., 19).

3 See Fraser Field, "Editorial," *The Vancouver Province*, 6 May 1996, 5.

4 See R. Röetzer, "The Sympto-Thermal Method: Ten Years of Change," *Lineacre Quarterly* 45 (1978): 358.

5 Probably the most widely used criterion used to recognize post-ovulatory infertility is the "coverline." This is a line drawn on the BBT graph 0.1 degree Fahrenheit above the last six low readings prior to the perceived rise. There must be three readings above the coverline to assure that post-ovulatory infertility has begun. Klaus, 9.

6 Ibid.

7 See Lyn Billings, "Teaching All Indicators Is Not the Same as Teaching All Methods—Some Clarifications," *Bulletin of the Ovulation Method Research and Reference Centre of Australia* (August 1994).

8 John J. Billings, *The Ovulation Method*, 7th ed. (Melbourne: Advocate Press, 1983).

9 Evelyn Billings and Ann Westmore, *The Billings Method*, 2nd ed. (Yarra, Victoria, Australia: Anne O'Donovan, Ltd, 1990).

10 Among Odeblad's published work, perhaps the most approachable is his appendix to Evelyn Billings, John Billings, and Maurice Catarinich, *Billings Atlas of the Ovulation Method*, 5th ed. (North Fitzroy, Victoria, Australia: Ovulation Method Research and Reference Center of Australia, 1989).

11 E. Billings et al., "Symptoms and Hormonal Changes Accompanying Ovulation," *Lancet* 1 (1972): 282–84.

12 T. Hilgers, G. Abraham, and D. Cavanagh, "The Peak Symptom and Estimated Time of Ovulation," *Natural Family Planning* 52 (November 1978): 5.

13 For example, see A. Jewell, "Unfair Burden on the Female Partner," *BMJ* 307 (1993): 1357. See also the lively discussion in the several issues of *BMJ* which followed Dr. Ryder's paper of 13 September 1993, referenced below.

14 G. Jarvis, "Empowers Couples," *BMJ* 307 (1993): 1358.

15 Klaus, 1.

16 J. Queenan et al., eds, "Natural Family Planning: Current Knowledge and New Strategies for the 1990s," Supplement to *American Journal of Obstetrics and Gynecology*, December 1991. This conference was co-sponsored by Georgetown University, the United States Agency for International Development, and the World Health Organization.

17 R. Ryder, "Natural Family Planning: Effective Birth Control Supported by the Catholic Church," *BMJ* 307 (1993): 723–26.

18 R. Ryder and H. Campbell, "Natural Family Planning in the 1990s," *Lancet*

346 (1995): 233–34.

[19] Billings and Westmore, ch. 16.

[20] Ibid.

[21] J. Trussell and L. Grummer-Strawn, "Further Analysis of Contraceptive Failure of the Ovulation Method," in Queenan, 2054–59.

[22] Ibid.

[23] A. Ghosh, cited in Ryder, *BMJ*, 725.

[24] M. Barbato and G. Bertolotti, "Natural Methods for Fertility Control: A Prospective Study," *Int J Fertility* 33 (1988): 48–51.

[25] See K. Severyn, "The Hidden Side of Norplant," *Linacre Quarterly* 62, no. 4 (November 1995): 59–66.

[26] Billings and Westmore, 79.

[27] Unless otherwise noted, all scriptural quotations in this article are taken from the New Revised Standard Version of the Bible, copyright the Division of Christian Education of the National Council of the Churches of Christ in the United States of America.

[28] Paul M. Quay, "Contraception and Conjugal Love," in *Why Humanae vitae Was Right*, ed. Janet E. Smith (San Francisco: Ignatius Press, 1993), 32–33.

[29] Ibid, 39.

[30] Dietrich von Hildebrand, "The Encyclical *Humanae vitae*: A Sign of Contradiction," in Smith, 79.

[31] Joseph Hattie, *Totally Yours* (London, On.: WOOMB Canada, 1993), 21.

[32] Charles D. Provan, *The Bible and Birth Control* (Monogahela, Penn.: Zimmer Printing, 1989), 63.

[33] Hattie, 22.

[34] *Humanae vitae*.

[35] Ruth Lassiter, "Sensible Sex," in Smith, 473–96.

[36] R. Patrick Homan, "Marital Chastity: A Blessing for Marriage, Family and Spiritual Life," in *Trust the Truth* (Braintree, Mass.: Pope John Center, 1991), 133–43.

[37] Lassiter, 479.

[38] Cormac Burke, "Marriage and Contraception," in Smith, 157.

[39] For instance, Jacqueline Kasun, *The War Against Population: The Economics and Ideology of Population Control* (San Francisco: Ignatius Press, 1988).

[40] *Humanae vitae*.

[41] At an address in Vancouver in November 1995, John Billings reported that the compulsory abortion policy was a major source of discontent in China and the government recognizes this. They have recruited the Billings to train NFP teachers there on a huge scale. One of the first groups that John and Lyn addressed were seventy-five female gynaecologists whose job was "pregnancy police": they had to seek out and abort any pregnant women who had already

borne a child. Some of these gynaecologists struck the Billings as heartless doctrinaire communists, but most of them seemed totally demoralized by their work.

42 Herbert F. Smith, "The Proliferation of Population Problems," in Smith, 398.

43 1970 commencement address at Smith College, quoted by Most Rev. Adam J. Maida, "Responsible Parenthood in the Writings of Pope John Paul II," *Linea-cre Quarterly* 55, no. 4 (November 1988): 26.

44 For helpful discussion on this issue, see *Humanae vitae* no. 10; Hattie, 44–49; and Janet E. Smith, "The Moral Use of Natural Family Planning" in Smith, 445–71.

45 *Humanae vitae* no. 21.

46 Janet E. Smith, "Pope John Paul II and *Humanae vitae*" in Smith, 233.

47 Elzbieta Wojcik, "Natural Regulation of Conception and Contraception" in Smith, 431; and Janet E. Smith, "*Humanae vitae* at Twenty" in Smith, 526.

48 Smith, ibid., 523.

49 Ibid.

50 Donald deMarco, "Abortion and Contraception," *Bulletin of the Ovulation Method Research and Reference Centre of Australia* 22, no. 1 (March 1995): 9–10.

51 John M. Haas, "Straight Talk About Contraception: The Church's 'Yes' to the Gift of Life" in *Trust the Truth*, 349.

52 Mary Rosera Joyce, "The Meaning of Contraception" in Smith, 115.

53 Joseph Boyle, "Contraception and Natural Family Planning" in Smith, 415.

54 Ibid., 417.

55 G. E. M. Anscombe, "Contraception and Chastity" in Smith, 123.

56 Ibid., 141–42.

57 Janet E. Smith, "Pope John Paul II and *Humanae vitae*," in Smith, 243.

Gerald L. Higgins

The Rise and Decline of Medical Professionalism and the Challenge to the Christian

Throughout the long history of medicine there are many examples of associations of healers of varied kinds, some founded upon a religious authority such as the healing cult of Aesklepios at Delphi, others based upon the charisma of a visionary healer, such as Hippocrates, while yet others erected their systems upon the explanatory power of theories such as those of the mathematician and mystic Pythagoras, from whose cult the Hippocratic Oath is believed to have been derived. There have also been associations of particular distinct types of healers who have been statutorily recognized and given various degrees of authority over other healers, such as the medieval divisions into the orders of physician, chirurgeon, and apothecary.

However, medicine—as a unified profession established by law and granted an exclusive monopoly to define the content of medicine, control entry, set educational standards, regulate practice, and discipline its members—came into being in Great Britain only about 150 years ago. Medical professionalism in the modern era arose out of conflict between various occupational groups who were concerned with the acquisition or maintenance of privilege and power, the dominance of or even exclusion of competing groups, and the entrenchment of a statutorily recognized monopoly of medical service. Such far-reaching changes took place during the contemporaneous social revolution which was marked by an unprecedented increase in population and a massive, innovative industrial production, and accompanied by a shift in political power from the aristocratic oligarchy of the landed interests to the manufacturing interests. At the same time, there was a massive expansion of medical knowledge which, with refinements of practice, seemed to confirm the value of rational enquiry and empirical experiment, attitudes arising out of the seventeenth-century Scientific Revolution and the eighteenth-century Enlightenment.

This evolution of a paradigmatic profession led to far-reaching changes. Nowadays many groups beyond the bounds of the health-care field, using similar techniques, have claimed formal recognition, often with legislated authority and corresponding financial rewards, all to be justified in the name of protection of the public. The very nature of the control of the social structure has changed, for as Perkins has noted, "professionalism permeates society from top to bottom," and, furthermore, "the professional hierarchies cut across the horizontal solidarities of class in the warp and weft of the social fabric."[1]

Today, however, in this postmodern era where science is no longer seen as the supreme arbiter, the atmosphere in which medicine is practised has changed from the adulatory acceptance of doctor pronouncements—as in the late nineteenth to the mid-twentieth century—to a severe doubt of its claims and a bitter criticism of its practices, while the individual authority of the doctor has been circumscribed by legal fiat, clinical guidelines, patient scepticism, and the shift from a physician paternalism to a contractual rights-based medicine.

The contemporary usage of the terms "profession" and "professional" has eroded the concept of what it means to be a member of a profession. In common usage, the term "professional" means little more than that one is paid for what one does, as, for example, we speak of a professional as opposed to an amateur athlete. It is also used to imply that a task has been well done as opposed to its being bungled, whether it be a bank robbery or a plumbing job. It may carry a derogatory flavour as when we say "professional politician," implying that the person so described makes a trade of what should be performed from higher motives. The term may even be used in a derisory sense when we speak of the "oldest profession."

In its core usage, the term denoted a declaration of one's belief and values. In medieval usage, it referred to the declaration made by postulants on their entry and commitment to a religious order, when they declared their beliefs, reasons, and goals in taking such a momentous step. The term was extended gradually to apply to the group which the individual entered, especially the three primary professions—divinity, law, and medicine—with an emphasis being placed on a vocational sense of service to God and man.

But why, how, where, and when at this particular period did the transformation of medicine take place? What motivated the reformers to persevere over such a lengthy period to persist with their efforts? What was wrong with the social organization of medicine and the character of medical practitioners that could impel them to such efforts?

The Eighteenth-Century Background

The period from the mid-eighteenth to the mid-nineteenth centuries was marked by intellectual ferment, revolutionary violence, war, technological change, and expanding overseas commerce and saw the end of the supremacy of landed privilege, the rise of the manufacturing interests, the reform of Parliamentary and local government, and the emergence of a society distinguished by self-conscious class status.

In the eighteenth century, England was a hierarchical society, characterized by fine gradations of status. At the apex of the hierarchical pyramid, a small and unified elite—the landed aristocracy—held within its hands the reigns of political, economic, and social power. The possession of property and the power of patronage were the essential means by which the triangular hierarchy of the social structure was maintained. There was one horizontal cleavage in this society, namely, that between the "gentleman" and the "common people." The fundamental requirement for the status of "gentleman" was an ability to support one's self without manual labour, to live on the income from property, and "included besides the nobility and gentry, the clergyman, physician, and barrister, but not always the Dissenting minister, the apothecary, the attorney, or the schoolmaster; the overseas merchant but not the inland trader; the amateur author, painter, musician but rarely the professional."[2] The concept of the "gentleman" required commitment to a "warrior" code, demanding bravery and skill at arms, together with the characteristics of courage, confidence, acceptance of obligation, and perseverance, honesty, and trustworthiness. As the emphasis on martial skills became less important, the requirement of fiscal resources to support the status and independence without manual or servile work remained, as did the expectation that the gentleman would adhere to the honour code of trustworthiness, honesty, fidelity, courage, and consideration for social inferiors.

Warfare was the one constant throughout the century, especially with France on the Continent, in North America, the West Indies, and India, a resultant of mercantile rivalry. The political expression of the beliefs in the "Rights of Man" and the consequent reactions resulted in the dialectic of violence, revolution, and repression as expressed in the American Revolution (1775-1883), the French Revolution (1789-1794), and the succeeding Napoleonic Wars, brought to an end by the bloody battle at Waterloo (1815).

The Philosophical and Religious Background

Intellectually, the Enlightenment philosophers in France, Britain, and Germany sought to replace what they designated as blind ignorance and superstition, fostered by religion, tradition, and hereditary privilege, with the light of certain and sure knowledge, garnered and directed by Reason, and evaluated by pragmatic experiment. They proclaimed the "Rights of Man," well expressed by Thomas Jefferson in his original draft of the American Declaration of Independence, that all men were "created equal and independent . . . with . . . rights inherent and inalienable, among which are the preservation of life, and liberty, and the pursuit of happiness."[3]

Immanuel Kant (1724-1804), the Konigsberg philosopher, son of a saddler, reputedly of Scots origin, reared in poverty and Pietism, sought to replace the religious and Christian basis for ethical behaviour with a philosophical basis in the "categorical imperative"—a secularized version of the Golden Rule—"Act only on that maxim through which you can at the same time will that it become universal law."[4]

Jeremy Bentham (1748-1832) expanded the concepts of pragmatism, rationality, empiricism, common sense, and scepticism—propounded earlier by Thomas Hobbes (1588-1679), John Locke

(1632-1704), Francis Hutcheson (1694-1746), and David Hume (1711-1776)—into a well-developed Utilitarianism. He proclaimed as axiomatic that the greatest good for the greatest number was the only true measure of right and wrong, and that the only ethical guide to evaluate proposed courses of action was the felicific calculus of pain and pleasure.

Bentham's associate, James Mill (1773-1836) and his son, John Stuart Mill (1806-1873), sought to develop both man and society in rational and empiric ways. These efforts culminated in the reform of Parliament with the Reform Bill of 1832, and the reorganization of local authorities and cities through the Hygiene and Sanitary Reform movement. This movement was an offshoot of Utilitarianism and initially directed by the lawyer and Poor Law reformer Edwin Chadwick (1801-1890), who had been Bentham's secretary. It also attracted physicians such as Thomas Southwood Smith (1788-1861) who gave the eulogy and performed the autopsy which constituted the burial service of Jeremy Bentham; the physician-statistician William Farr (1807-1883); and the surgeon-reformer Sir John Simon (1816-1904).

The rationalistic temper of philosophical thought dismissed religious belief as at best, misguided sentiment, or even worse as a dangerous delusion from which one must be delivered. The established Anglican church, characterized by a cold rationalistic faith, was regarded merely as a powerful instrument for safeguarding the interests of the reigning political party, and to provide "livings" for younger sons of the gentry and nobility. Dissent, heir of the sixteenth-century Puritan revolution, was inturned, if not moribund, and failed to meet the needs of the masses in the new towns. There was, nonetheless, a dynamic re-awakening of Christian faith, especially among the common people of Great Britain and the Thirteen Colonies. The Evangelical movement, arising out the work of the brothers John and Charles Wesley and of George Whitfield, and forced into a separatist mode by the implacable hostility of the Anglican hierarchy, revitalized the ranks of Dissent, but without the political radicalism of Puritanism. The vigorous drive for an active, selfless Christian life with an emphasis on thrift, abstinence, and hard work led to the development of a cohesive movement in which the dispossessed and alienated could once again meet a need for fulfilment and power, based on their personal redemption through the death and resurrection of a transcendent, yet immanent, Saviour. Together with the evangelical Anglican group, the influential Clapham Sect under the leadership of William Wilberforce (1759-1833), there was a long-sustained movement for the abolition of slavery, first in the United Kingdom in 1807, and later abroad. The legislation that led to the amelioration of the savage exploitation of women and children in the "dark, Satanic mills"—William Blake's (1757-1827) description—of the expanding factories and mines of the early Industrial Revolution was introduced by Wilberforce's successor as leader of the Clapham Sect, Lord Anthony Ashley Cooper, seventh Earl of Shaftesbury (1801-1885), with the Coal Mine Act (1842) which prohibited the employment underground of women and children under thirteen years of age, and the Factory Acts of 1847 and 1850 which reduced the hours of exploitative labour in the new factories.

The Population Expansion; the Agricultural and Industrial Transformation
This same period was marked also by a massive fourfold increase in the population. The population of England and Wales seems to have been virtually stagnant in the first four decades of the century at about 5.8 to 6 million people. Over the next century, the rate of population growth increased to such a degree that by 1861, the population of England and Wales had reached just over twenty-three million.[5]

The introduction of new techniques of agricultural production, introduced by men such as Jethro Tull, "Turnip" Townshend, and Coke of Holkham, led to a contemporaneous agrarian revolution with a large increase in home-grown foods sufficient to feed the expanding population with little food import. However, these agrarian improvements were accompanied by a massive land enclosure and displacement of the peasantry, "divorced from the land, owning no means of production, often workless as well as landless."[6]

The concomitant industrial revolution made possible by the development of steam power and the invention of machines to do work previously requiring skilled workers, the availability of cheap labour, displaced by the enclosures as well as Irish immigration, with a rising population, led to an increase in output per head and in the gross national product. These demographic, agrarian, and industrial changes led to a large scale urbanization with a great increase in the size and numbers of manufacturing towns. It was a world where child labour was systematically exploited as never before, for children were easy to discipline both to the repetitive operations required by the machine as well as to the harsh routine of the long factory hours; and with a rising population they were readily available and cheap. William Wordsworth (1770–1850) described the scenes of factory life in his poem, *The Excursion*, published in 1814.

> Men, maidens, youths,
> Mother and little children, boys and girls,
> Enter, and each the wonted task resumes
> Within this temple, where is offered up
> To Gain, the master-idol of the realm,
> Perpetual sacrifice.[7]

A concomitant steady inflation eroded any gains in income made by workers and farm labourers. It has been estimated that the price of a typical basket of consumer goods rose nearly 40% in the period 1760 to 1792, with a further doubling of prices between 1793 and 1815—the whole period being one of almost continuous warfare.[8]

These changes were not without their effect upon the health of the people in the new industrial cities. Edwin Chadwick (1800–1890), Secretary of the Sanitary Commission (1839), appointed a committee to study the London districts with the highest typhus mortality: in their Report of 1838, they revealed the full squalor of the London rookeries.[10] A few years later, in 1842, he published the *Report on the Sanitary Conditions of the Labouring Population* which in-

Location	Gentry, Professional People, Avg. Age of Death (No. of deaths)	Tradesmen, Farmers, Shopkeepers Avg. Age of Death (No. of Deaths)	Mechanics & Labourers Avg. Age of Death (No. of Deaths)
County of Rutland	52	41	38
Liverpool	35 (137)	22 (1,738)	15 (5,597)
Leeds	44 (79)	27 (824)	19 (3,395)
Bethnal Green, London	45 (101)	26 (237)	16 (1,258)

Table I. Expectation of Years of Life according to occupation and place.[9]

cluded some startling observations on the expectation of life in various parts of the country in relation to social status and occupation.

The Emergence of Economic Theory

Alongside these changes there was also a rapid evolution of a free market system and capitalism, with joint stock companies with limited liability and an expanded banking system. A discipline of political economy that sought to explain and justify these rapid social changes emerged from the work of Adam Smith (1723–1790), Thomas Malthus (1766–1834), and David Ricardo (1772–1823). The belief that the unfettered operation of the market, under the "invisible hand" (Adam Smith's phrase) of an economic providence, could provide the best of all possible worlds was a politico-economic expression of the rationalistic Deism characteristic of the age. Alexander Pope (1688–1744), the lame but dominant poetic genius of the era, in his *Essay on Man*, described the underlying reductionist philosophy.

> All Nature is but art, unknown to thee,
> All chance, direction, which thou canst not see;
> All discord, harmony not understood;
> All partial evil, universal good;
> And, spite of pride, in erring reason's spite,
> One truth is clear, Whatever is, is right.[11]

Such beliefs, replacing the older hierarchical "great chain of being" in which everyone had duties and obligations to those above and below them, justified in rationalistic terms the vast discrepancy of wealth, power, and rank, and was used to exploit the less fortunate within the society, as well as to sanction the cruelty, brutality, and indifference of the age to suffering. The "trickle-down" theory of economics, used to justify the greed and lavish excesses of the Reagan era in the United States, was also described by Alexander Pope. In his *Moral Essays*, the narrator, after a lavish banquet, declared:

> Treated, caress'd, and tired, I take my leave,
> Sick of his civil pride from morn to eve;
> Curse such lavish cost and little skill
> And swear no day was passed so ill.
> Yet hence the poor are clothed, the hungry fed;
> Health to himself, and to his infant's bread,

> The labourer bears: what his hard heart denies,
>   His charitable vanity supplies."[12]

The "hard heart" refers not to the labourer, but to the giver of the sumptuous banquet! Such beliefs were used to justify an individualism which was at a radical variance to the Christian belief that one had a duty to one's neighbour to love the neighbour as one's self.

Radical Responses and Repressive Reaction

These changes—intellectual, social, economic, and demographic—together with technical innovation, ushered in a century of social and political upheaval accompanied by a sometimes violent agitation for change, leading to a savage repression through the Anti-Combination Acts of 1799–1800 which made it illegal to "combine" to get higher wages, better working conditions, attend meetings, or raise funds. Despite these various repressive Acts, active protest was demonstrated by the Luddite destruction of machinery (1811–1813), the Spa Field Riots in London in 1816, an attack on the Prince Regent's carriage after the opening of Parliament in 1817, the Peterloo massacre in Birmingham in 1819, the Cato Street Conspiracy to kill members of the Cabinet as they dined with the Prime Minister in 1820, and the burning of hay-ricks and barns by "Captain Swing" in 1830–31. The Chartist movement sought universal adult suffrage, a secret ballot, and compulsory universal education. In general it was non-violent, but on occasion the movement resorted to conspiracy, sedition, and rebellion such as the ineffectual rebellion of 1839 in South Wales and the Birmingham Bull Ring Riots the same year,[13] while in 1842 there were the "plug riots" in which Lancashire workers demanded the restoration of the 1840 wage levels. There was a savage repression, with suspension of *Habeas Corpus*, and the passage of the infamous Six Acts, leading to an almost complete suspension of the Constitution. Many were sentenced to imprisonment and transportation to the then penal colony of Australia, while others were executed.

Medicine in the Late Eighteenth and Early Nineteenth Centuries

The late eighteenth and early nineteenth centuries saw a transformation of medicine in terms of its knowledge base, techniques, organization, numbers, and social prestige. At the start of the period, it was characterized by its medieval organization, its knowledge base related to the ancient concepts of humoral homeostasis, and its practice dependent on blood-letting and herbs known to the ancients. By the end of the period, the profession was unified with formal registration and supervision, with a knowledge base founded on morbid anatomical science, a clinical methodology, an early laboratory science, an understanding of hygiene and the role of bacterial infection, as well as the rudimentary beginnings of modern therapeutics.

The Practitioners of Medicine

The social organization of medicine was that inherited from the Middle Ages: namely, the division into three distinct groups, diverse as to their historic origin, social status, education, field of practice, and income. "Between the physician, who could claim to belong to a learned profession, the surgeon who practised a craft, and the apothecary who followed a trade, the gap was wide and impassable."[14] This division was rigid and hierarchical with "its ranks and orders, each with own function and sphere of usefulness; and each estate had its necessary position of subordination and authority."[15] Between the elite of university educated practitioners and apprenticeship and private medical school trained doctors there was "an extraordinary degree of bitterness and hostility."[16]

Vocational stratification was rigid in the eighteenth century—membership of each group was exclusive. Entry into one group precluded membership of another, or required relinquishment of an existing membership. However, the reality was that many physicians, with university degrees, especially with Scottish qualifications, practised surgery, midwifery, and prescribed medicines, while many surgeons saw "as many patients in the character of a physician, as of a surgeon."[17]

Medical practitioners were not regarded with any great respect as the contemporary novelists and diarists demonstrate. They were regarded as venal and corrupt. Benjamin Rush (1745–1813), an American physician, reformer, and signer of the American Declaration of Independence, who obtained his MD in 1768 from Edinburgh, noted that the doctors of his day, in their relation towards patients, were often guilty of falsehood, inhumanity, avarice, and neglect.[18] Relationships between members of the tripartite division of medicine were often acrimonious and bitter, including duelling,[19] and were not ameliorated by pamphlet wars between individual practitioners.[20] From Chaucer onwards to Smollett, Fielding, and Richardson in the eighteenth century, the image of medical practitioners more often emphasised their rapacity and exploitative pomposity rather than their compassion and competence. It was not until later—with Jane Austen, Anthony Trollope, and George Eliot—that the practitioners of medicine began to be presented in a more favourable light.

The Physicians

At the apex of the hierarchy were the physicians, i.e., Fellows or licentiates of the Royal College of Physicians of London (1518) or the similar colleges of Edinburgh and Dublin, established in the seventeenth century, or graduates with degrees in physic from the ancient Universities of Oxford and Cambridge. They were drawn from the ranks of the gentry, with a prolonged university education in which they studied the classics of medicine, Hippocrates, Galen, and their commentators. They had little bedside training—at the beginning of our period few hospitals existed—and the anatomical requirements of their training would be met by observing dissections of executed criminals. Their clinical education was pursued in the medical schools of France and Holland.

The Surgeons

Below physicians in the social hierarchy, the surgeons were considered as tradesmen of inferior degree who used the servants' entrance. Often, they were less well educated in terms of a formal university education, but were prepared with a great deal of practical experience and were engaged in a brutal and bloody branch of the healing art. As early as 1387, a craft guild of barbers was formed and some of its members practised a primitive surgery. The association between barbers and surgeons continued somewhat uneasily, despite the formation in 1540 of the Barber-Surgeons Company of the City of London. Their divorce occurred in 1745 when the Company of Surgeons of the City of London was founded; in 1800, the Company became the Royal College of Surgeons of London and in 1843 was granted status as the Royal College of Surgeons of England. Despite their inferior social status, considerable developments in both the theory and practice of the "craft" had taken place as a result of the work of the Hunter brothers, William and John, and other surgeons of the period.

The Apothecaries

Inferior to both physicians and surgeons, the apothecaries in their origins were associated with mercers, grocers, spicers, and pepperers in the craft-guild of the Grocers' Company. In a 1540 Act of Parliament, they were given a special status within that Company, being referred to as the "mystery of apothecaries." In 1617, under a charter granted by James I, the Society of Apothecaries was founded, giving a degree of respectability to the apothecary. In 1704, the conviction of an apothecary for illegal practice of medicine was overturned on appeal to the House of Lords. Apothecaries did not charge for their advice and services but simply for the medicines that they prescribed, confirming a general perception of the apothecary as being a small trader rather than a member of an educated profession. In 1829 a judge, Lord Tenterden, in the Handey v. Hanson case, decided that an apothecary could in fact charge for his attendance rather than "sending large and useless quantities of medicine."[21]

In the last two decades of the eighteenth century, the "chemist and druggist" began to dispense drugs and medicines much more cheaply than the apothecary and threatened their livelihood. The chemists and druggists were openly supported by the physicians who were thus freed from dependence upon the apothecary.

The New Practitioners—General Practitioners and Scottish MDs

General practitioners were a new type of practitioner who cut across the traditional tripartite division, for they practised medicine, surgery, and obstetrics as well as dispensed medicines. Their training was usually through an apprenticeship supplemented by study at private medical schools in London, as well as walking the wards of London hospitals, and confirmed by the possession of the diploma of membership of the Royal College of Surgeons. They found ready employment in the navy and military forces during the Napoleonic Wars. There also began to be a change in their occupation—arising out of the work of Sir John Pringle (1707–1782) and Captain James

Cook (1728–1779)—from a purely curative role, whether medical or surgical, to more of a social control model in the prevention of outbreaks of infectious disease in institutions whether gaols, hospitals, or naval vessels.

Alternative Practitioners of Medicine

For a large part of the population during this period, and for long after until a state insured health service was introduced, the bulk of medical care was provided by others than formally recognized practitioners, such as the village blacksmith, barber, herbalist, druggist, bone-setter, or midwife, and whose fees were much lower, often in-kind, and with whom the formally recognized medical practitioner had to compete.[22] In 1806, one physician, Edward Harrison, published the results of his survey of health care practitioners in rural Lancashire, showing that of all those in practice, physicians constituted only 2% of all healers, surgeons and apothecaries 9%, druggists 16%, and irregular practitioners and midwives 73%.[23]

Comparison of the results of the 1851 Census for England and Wales with the Medical Directory demonstrate that the former showed a total of 28,315 practitioners, both qualified and unqualified, but not distinguished into categories, while the Directory showed a total of 10,130 qualified practitioners, i.e., a discrepancy that suggests there were 18,185 unqualified practitioners in England and Wales![24] In the absence of any system of formal education, registration, and licensing, there was no decisive clarifying distinction between the orthodox regular practitioner and the unorthodox irregular practitioner.

The authoritative medical and surgical texts of the day were not the sole preserve of the medical establishment, for they formed part of the literature of the elite and middling classes, not only as cultural icons but also as practical resources for those who had servants, labourers, and other dependants. William Buchan (1729–1805) published his *Domestic Medicine* for that very purpose, and was subjected to severe criticism by the faculty for so doing.[25] Another popular source of information for the literate layman was John Wesley's *Primitive Physic*, first published in 1747; it was immensely popular and by 1840 had gone through thirty-six editions (my own copy was published in 1958!). Wesley wrote that "It is my design to set down cheap and safe and easy medicines, easily to be known, easy to be procured, and easy to be applied by plain, unlettered men."[26] Thomas Turner (1729–1793), a grocer in Sussex, had an extensive collection of medical books which he used in his role of caring for the poor as parish overseer.[27]

The Market of Medicine

Patronage, the major mechanism of social control in the eighteenth century, not only extended to the social status of physicians but also to their attitudes and beliefs, for medical knowledge was accessible to any educated person.[28] Aristocratic approbation could initiate treatments of which physicians disapproved, as, for example, Lady Mary Wortly Montagu's promotion of smallpox inoculation in 1722, based on observations of Turkish practice when she accompanied her husband as British Consul to the Ottoman Caliphate. Her motivation and enthusiasm for prevention of smallpox lay in the fact that she herself had suffered severe facial scarring as a result of her own bout with smallpox.[29]

Medical practice in a patronage system of medicine was controlled by the interest of the patient rather than by the knowledge and authority of the doctor, and as a result it was oriented to the relief of symptoms rather than the diagnosis of disease. The patron, as patient, could define not only the nature of the illness but also dictate the programme of medicine as being directed to the relief of symptoms rather than the diagnosis, investigation, and treatment of disease.[30]

In general, the medical market prior to the Industrial Revolution was limited and uncertain, and savage competition was common. Poverty was the lot of many of practitioners, while others supplemented their income by engaging in retail trade, a practice that continued well into the nineteenth century.[31] However as the Great Transformation took place, with industrialization and urbanization and a massive increase in the population, there was an increase in the medical market, and it became easier for recognized practitioners to become established.[32]

The Transformation of Medicine

The transformation of medicine was produced by a number of factors, including a concern about the behaviour of practitioners and the development of ethical codes; the development of the hospital; the rise of medical schools; the expansion of medical knowledge, technology, and theory; together with the emergence of vigorous local and specialized societies dedicated to medical reform. These changes culminated in the Apothecaries' Act of 1815, the reorganization of the London College of Surgeons in 1843, and the Medical Acts of 1851 and 1886.

The Development of Professional Codes of Ethics

Doctors were well aware of the derision, doubt, and suspicion with which the public regarded them and, as a result, made conscious attempts to improve their public image. John Gregory (1724-1773), Professor of Medicine at Edinburgh, in his *Lectures on the Duties and Qualifications of Physician*, 1772, commented that

> ridicule has rather been employed against physicians than physik. There are some reasons for this sufficiently obvious. Physicians considered as a body of men, have an interest separate and distinct from the honour of the science. In pursuit of this interest, some have acted with candour, with honour, in the ingenous and liberal manners of a gentleman. Conscious of their own worth, they disdained every artifice and depended for success on their real merit. But such men are most numerous in any profession. Some compelled by necessity, some stimulated by vanity, and others anxious to conceal ignorance, have had recourse to various mean and unworthy arts to raise their importance among the ignorant, who are always the numerous part of mankind. Some of these arts have been an affectation of mystery in all their writings and conversations relating to their profession; an affectation of knowledge, inscrutable to all, except the adepts in their science; an air of perfect confidence in their own skill and abilities; and a demeanour solemn, contemptuous, and highly expressive of self-sufficiency. These arts, however they might have served with the rest of mankind, could not escape the censure of the more judicious, nor evade the ridicule of

the men of wit and humour.[33]

He also noted that

the quarrels of physicians, when they end in appeals to the public, generally hurt the contending parties; but what is of more consequence, they discredit the profession, and expose the faculty itself to redicule and contempt.[34]

He also described medicine

as a liberal profession, whose object is the life and health of the human species, a profession to be exercised by gentlemen of honour and ingenuous manners; the dignity of which can never be supported by means that are inconsistent with its ultimate object, and that only tends to increase the pride and fill the pockets of a few individuals.[35]

Earlier in his lectures, he had commented that

besides the good which a physician has it often in his power to do, in consequence of skill in his profession, there are many occasions that call for assistance as a man who feels for the misfortunes of his fellow creatures. In this respect, he has many opportunities of displaying patience, good-nature, generosity, compassion, and all the gentler virtues that do honour to the human condition.[36]

The book by Thomas Percival (1740–1804) published posthumously in 1803, entitled *Medical Ethics: A Code of Institutes and Precepts Adopted to the Professional Conduct of Physicians and Surgeons* is largely concerned with promoting harmonious relationships between physicians, surgeons, and apothecaries at the Manchester Royal Infirmary. These relationships were strained by the stress of dealing with a typhus epidemic in 1789, and aggravated by the actions of the trustees of the hospital who without consulting the existing staff, appointed more medical staff, and by so doing created conflict. Percival's principal goal was, in his own words,

to promote the honour and advancement of his profession . . . to frame a general system of medical ethics; that the official conduct and mutual intercourse of the faculty might be regulated by precise and acknowledged

principles of urbanity and rectitude.[37]
In the same vein as Gregory, Percival wrote in the dedication of the book to his son, that

> the study of professional Ethics, therefore cannot fail to invigorate and enlarge your understanding; whilst the observance of the duties which they enjoin, will soften your manners, expand your affections, and form you to that propriety and dignity of conduct, which are essential to the character of a *gentleman*.[38]

In 1814, R. M. Kerrison published an account of the medical profession and described the kind of man a medical practitioner was expected to be.

> The medical character, whether Physician, Surgeon, or Prescribing Apothecary, should be a man of integrity, urbanity, and sedateness, patient of fatigue, and ever ready to extend the beneficial influence of his art upon principles of enlarged philanthropy; he must necessarily sustain many privations of comfort and of rest by the sudden and urgent calls to administer relief, and, indeed, to be extensively useful, he must often indulge his better feelings at the expense of his convenience, by affording assistance, without the hope, or expectation of a pecuniary reward.[39]

Another physician, writing somewhat later in 1837, could say that

> we should not . . . be exposed to feel or witness, or even hear of those feuds, which sometimes arise between members of the profession, so injurious to the interest of all concerned, and so derogatory to that high character, which it is our duty to preserve, and should be our chief aim to raise in the estimation of the public.[40]

These manuals of ethical codes and exhortations for gentlemanly behaviour were a deliberate attempt to increase the public stature of doctors with the ultimate goal of securing a sufficient standing to ensure legislative approval of a favoured and protected status. These ideals and attitudes of moral responsibility and personal trustworthiness were promoted through the development of a professional *mores*, expressive of the values and norms of doctors as a group, and formulated through ethical codes by which the boundaries of appropriate physician behaviour should be demarcated. All medical practitioners, through their individual personal behaviour, were exhorted to promote "the high character of the profession . . . and aim to raise [it] in the estimation of the public."[41]

The Development of Hospitals

The development of the charitable hospitals, commencing in the eighteenth century, first in London and Edinburgh and the major provincial cities, and expanding throughout the country in the nineteenth century, was an expression of concern over the state of the indigent, homeless, and poverty stricken who became ill. They were staffed by unpaid physicians and surgeons who attended those patrons with the power and wealth to establish such institutions and the honorary consulting staff, as they were called, received public recognition and acquired privilege and power as a consequence of their association with the institution and the wealthy.

As medical and particularly surgical knowledge and practice expanded, the hospitals became medical workplaces rather than custodial institutions, and effective governance passed to the medical staff, dominated largely by surgeons whose craft was becoming increasingly effective. The relationship towards patients also changed, for as the hospital staff were of a higher status socially, educationally, and economically than the patients whom they treated in these institutions, there was a shift in the power balance in the doctor's advantage, as opposed to their dependency in a patronage relationship.

The Rise of Medical Schools

One feature of the eighteenth-century medical scene was the emergence in London and the major provincial cities of private anatomical and medical academies, such as that of the Hunter brothers, William and John (1728–1793), which operated from 1746 to 1833. These schools, established by the entrepreneurial enterprise of the staff of the voluntary hospitals, were associated with the hospital and reflected the demand for doctors and their services, a demand created not only by the population expansion, but also by the increasing wealth of the population.

Students attending these schools had already completed their apprenticeship and were walking the wards for the required six months before their licensing examination, and many resented the compulsion inherent in the Apothecaries' Act, 1815.[42] These young men from the provinces and county towns, now in London, away from family and supervision, regarded the six months as a holiday before entering the hard and demanding life of the apothecary. "Little wonder that they became notorious as the wildest set in town, drunken, lecherous, making the night hideous with their pandemonium,"[43] immortalized by Charles Dickens with his bibulous, hearty character, Bob Sawyer, in *Pickwick Papers*, published in 1836.

Apprenticeship, with its personal relationship with an individual master, was gradually replaced by a medical education that was a formalized and centralized experience shared in common by students under the direction of the consulting specialists of the teaching hospitals. This educational process, removed from practise within the community, and centred exclusively in the teaching hospital, created a professional seclusion in which socialization to the values, beliefs, and professional practices of the medical elites could readily occur alongside formal medical education, creating a particular sense of a medical identity as well as a common professional ethos.

The Expansion of Medical Knowledge

During this period, from the late eighteenth to the late nineteenth centuries, there was a rapid expansion of clinical knowledge in the fields of obstetrics, surgery, and preventive medicine (including military hygiene and the prevention of scurvy and smallpox), leading to a painless antiseptic surgery, a relatively painless and safer obstetrics, a recognition and prevention of infectious diseases, as well as the recognition of specific disease syndromes associated with the suprarenal and thyroid glands and kidney. The old Hippocratic tradition—the balance of the four humours, the four primary opposites (hot and cold, wet and dry), the influence of climate and diet—which had survived for some two millennia was transformed into the critical knowledge-based experimental medicine with which we are familiar. Patients were transformed from the role as "subject" to that of "object" of detached scientific curiosity and observation by the doctor, an approach which was empirical, founded upon clinical evidence, based on technologically-supported data and subjected to evaluation and verification by post-mortem studies.

Contributing to this expansion of clinical knowledge was the development of an ever-expanding technology of medicine, associated at first with the minute and seconds watch, stethoscope, ophthalmoscope, thermometer, and sphygmomanometer; supplemented by laboratory studies and the discovery of X-rays later in the nineteenth century.

Medical knowledge was disseminated in journals such as *The Gentleman's Magazine*, more for the enlightenment of the layperson than the development of the technical competence of the doctor. A professional literature designed solely for the medical practitioner developed, with journals such as the *Lancet*, founded in 1823 by the surgeon-reformer Thomas Wakley (1795–1862), and the *British Medical Journal* of 1840, preceded by a quarterly, *The Midland Medical and Surgical Reporter* of 1828.

The Process of Medical Reform

At the end of the eighteenth century and the first half of the nineteenth centuries, there was much dissatisfaction with the existing social structure of medicine, especially among the apothecaries, so much so that they engaged in movements directed at reorganization of the formal structures of medicine for some seventy years.

The Apothecaries' Act 1815

The apothecaries were well aware of their marginal and lowly status and sought formal legitimation and recognition, and after some twenty years of agitation the Apothecaries Act, 1815, was finally passed. This was "an Act designed by the medical colleges for their suppression [of apothecaries], and administered by a Society not fit for the purpose," for they had fallen "into the hands of elderly men with little or no knowledge of clinical practice, but considerable expertise in nepotism."[44] The Society of Apothecaries of London was a livery company, a mercantile organization concerned with the import of drugs and spices rather than with the emerging science-based medicine and the care of patients and was a cynical move by the senior Colleges to maintain their status, privilege, and dominance.

However, the Act did establish over the United Kingdom a requirement for licensure by the Society of Apothecaries, and estab-

lished not so much an educational control of the required apprenticeship, as an exit evaluation of the apprenticeship before registration with and membership of the Society could be undertaken.
Membership of the Society, was achieved by examination, and required certificated evidence of attendance of lectures on anatomy,
botany, chemistry, materia medica, and the theory and practice of
physic, with six months work in a hospital, infirmary, or dispensary.
By the same token, apprenticeship as the means of entry retained
the tradesman status of the apothecary in a period when trade was
considered to be an inferior if not debased occupation.

Reform after the 1815 Apothecaries' Act

After the passage of the 1815 Apothecaries' Act and despite the
sense of betrayal and disappointment that many apothecaries and
general practitioners felt, efforts continued to improve the lot of the
general practitioner both in terms of medical knowledge as well as
status. The continued impetus for medical reform came from the
younger practitioners who were vigorous, militant agitators for reform: men such as Thomas Wakley, who founded the *Lancet* in
1823, and Charles Hastings, who resurrected the Worcester Medical
and Surgical Society in 1816 and transformed it into the Provincial
Medical and Surgical Association in 1832 (it became the British
Medical Association in 1855). It admitted all levels of recognized
practitioners and, in addition to its political goals, sought to promote medical knowledge by publishing various journals, culminating
in the *British Medical Journal* in 1857.

Surgical Reform—The Royal College of Surgeons of England, 1843

Much of the activity of the general practitioner reformers was directed at the College of Surgeons of London, for they believed that
it would represent them as full members. In 1843 the new charter,
which reconstituted the London College of Surgeons as the Royal
College of Surgeons of England and introduced a new rank of Fellowship, also ensured that it became responsible for the control of
surgical practice throughout the kingdom. The new Royal College of
Surgeons was governed, not by the old self-perpetuating oligopoly
but by a Council, elected by the new Fellows, some three hundred in
number who were selected from the leading surgeons of the day. Fel-

lows subsequently were acquired by examination, the first examination being in 1844 when twenty-four candidates passed.[45] The general practitioners, as being merely members of the College, were excluded from voting and from any part of running the College and policy decision-making.

The Medical Acts of 1858 and 1866

A number of Acts were introduced to regulate the medical profession, the first in 1840 and the sixteenth, and finally successful one, in 1858. However, the Act did not abolish the multiple portals of entry to medicine; neither, in the climate of *laissez-faire*, did it abolish quackery and unregistered practitioners, nor did it control medical education, although it could influence it by withholding approval of medical teaching institutions. The General Medical Council was heavily weighted in its membership towards the three medical corporations, especially the Royal Colleges. Furthermore, the Act perpetuated the recognition of the partially qualified doctor, for it was not until the 1886 Amendment Act that licensure required qualification in medicine, surgery, and midwifery. Only to a minor degree did the Act foster a corporate identity—a common purpose and pride, based on a common entrance and education—and it confirmed the inferior status of the general practitioner.

The General Council on Medical Education and Registration, familiarly known as the General Medical Council, "established the institutional basis of the modern structure of professional self regulation . . . to regulate the profession on behalf of the state, to oversee medical education, and to maintain a register of qualified practitioners."[46] The Council was given formal powers to discipline practitioners—even to remove names from the register—for sexual misconduct with patients, blatant advertising, and misrepresentation; this led to a compulsory acceptance of, rather than a purely voluntary adherence to, a minimal standard of a common code of ethical behaviour. By the same token, this dependency upon a statutorily based General Medical Council for professional recognition reduced the dependency upon lay patronage and validation.

The 1858 Medical Act did not create a medical monopoly, for it did not outlaw unorthodox practitioners such as herbalists, homeopaths, or those with deviant medical cosmologies. This did not occur until the 1886 revision of the Act. The medical market was still open and patients were free to consult whom they wished. The Act provided that only properly qualified doctors could be appointed to the burgeoning numbers of public posts that were being created in the poor-law medical services, public health service, colonial medical services, prison service, insane asylums, or the armed forces.[47]

Achievement of Professionalism: Professional and Social Recognition

Surgeons and apothecaries were regarded merely as tradesmen of inferior status rather than as members of a learned profession. They sought social status, for many of them were marginalized; and they also sought legitimation, for an important source of medical practitioner discontent was competition from unrecognized practitioners, a discontent predicated on at least two grounds. The first of these was the risk of harm that the unrecognized practitioner represented to the public. They also sought protection from competition by means of a legitimated medical monopoly on the ground that "medical education was an investment and that unqualified practitioners were denying those who were qualified a legitimate return on that investment."[48] They sought power to control medical education and to pronounce authoritatively on matters of medical importance.

The status and power, the charisma, of the doctor would no longer solely be a matter of personal endowment or achievement, but would be supplemented by that of a group whose mantle would be thrown over the individual doctor, endowing him with an authority to pronounce the powerful incantation, "In my professional opinion . . . ."

The achievement of status for the modern profession resulted in

1. an independence from lay control of medical decisionmaking, i.e., an end to the patronage system of medicine;
2. the ability to control the nature and content of vocational activity;
3. an exclusivity of medical services defined by the profession and a monopoly of medical services defined by statute, certification of birth and death.

The justifications that the medical reformers used to support their claims for statutory legitimation were fourfold, namely,

1. the increasing inaccessibility of medical scientific knowledge

to the lay person, together with an increasing therapeutic effectiveness;

2. the control of competence and the protection of the public from the risk of harm by untrained, unscientific, exploitative alternative practitioners;

3. the claim of a primacy of an ethic of service to the patient and public;

4. the trustworthiness of practitioners as men of honour.

The end result of the development of a full-fledged professionalism was that doctors were members of a professionally educated elite, members of a state-approved hierarchy founded on the certain knowledge of science, authorized to pronounce on life and death and with the exclusive right to prescribe powerful and dangerous drugs. The power differentiation between doctor and patient, a discrepancy enforced by the dependency of sickness, was now reinforced by statutory legitimation and authority, professional independence, and a recognized social status.

The motivations that lay behind the drive of nineteenth century medical practitioners to achieve recognition and legitimation through legislation were complex, a mixture of self-serving pragmatic opportunism and altruistic idealism, for they sought, to use that quintessential Victorian expression, "respectability," expressed in terms of social status and fiscal reward. The emphasis that the medical reformers, Gregory and Percival, placed upon the desirability of the aristocratic status of a gentleman for the doctor was not so much on the possession of wealth to ensure independence, but on the demonstration of a character marked by integrity, honesty, trustworthiness, the recognition and acceptance of obligation, a generosity of spirit, and on the adherence to a code of conduct which included being considerate of women and children and being polite and courteous to all. These were virtues not only for the privileged physician, many of whom came from the ranks of the gentry, but for all who aspired to be formally recognized as "healers." In the industrial era, the social ideal was that of the entrepreneur who, with capital, would utilize new ideas to develop a business, and the medical man of the nineteenth century, though still required to possess the values, attitudes, and behaviours of the "gentleman," was also to be ready to adopt new ideas, develop new techniques, and advance the pursuit of knowledge.

If the gentleman-doctor, in addition to possessing a virtuous character, could afford to be independent and hence, impartial and disinterested; and if the entrepreneurial-doctor was to be aggressive in the pursuit of knowledge and its applications; what were the distinguishing features of the doctor in the era of professionalism? They were a prolonged formal training, certified expertise, and professional success based upon merit. These characteristics of professional membership enabled one to "rent out" an expertise, where the fees charged related not only to the actual service provided but also reflected the costs of the acquisition and certification of that expertise as well as the scarcity value resulting from monopoly.

In our day—postmodern and dominated by the ideology of a free market, with legal fiat and fiscal management as the dominant and controlling ideologies—the over-riding social ideal is the acquisition of wealth and privileged status arising from media recognition.

The Decline of Professionalism

Although the nominal status quo of the profession of medicine has remained unchanged, there have been significant changes since the Second World War that have eroded the independence, status, and power of the profession.

The emergence of both tax-supported and privately managed health-care systems, together with the development of a high-technology medicine, have had significant effects on the status of the profession. Physicians in both state-funded and privately managed health-care systems, although still nominally independent practitioners, have in effect become functionaries, remunerated and subjected to fiscal and practice surveillance by government and business bureaucracies. Within the supervising bureaucracies of both government and business, medicine has been displaced from its previous centrality with a resulting loss of influence, as now it is but another special interest group whose advice may be disregarded without too much consequence.

A number of factors have led to this erosion in the status, power, and influence of the profession. Among them are the development of a high-technology medicine, the emergence of an administrative controlling bureaucracy, the rise of feminism, the diffusion of technical knowledge and the emergence of consumerism, the rise of bio-ethics and the shift in the ethical basis of medicine, the increased scrutiny of the profession and the revelations of physician malpractice and exploitation.

It is ironic that the very successes of medicine as scientifically based and technologically advanced have contributed to the devaluing of doctors. The increasingly technological nature of medicine has led to a distancing and detachment of the doctor from the patient as a person. The patient is an object of scientific gaze that is detached, objective, and dispassionate and is not very concerned with the fears, hopes, dreams, and desires of the patient that have been threatened if not shattered by the onset of the illness. Associated with this is the belief that medicine can now "cure" disease, that is transform and correct the process that has led to the emergence of the illness, whereas the doctor of previous eras, could, at the most, only interfere with the process and relieve symptoms.[49] The demand for standardization and conformity of treatment has transformed the role of the physician from that of an artist, free to choose and act creatively, to that of a labourer carrying out the dictates of a master.[50] The image of the doctor is that of the white-coated scientist-engineer rather than that of a beneficent father-figure healer.

The emergence of a hospital medicine, based on high-cost technology, has led to the development of massive bureaucracies as a result of the demand for substantial funding, efficiency, and control. In turn, together with the disinterest of doctors in medical-institutional administration, this has led to the development of a new profession, that of health-care administration. The administration of major hospitals and, indeed, all the institutions of the public sector, is shaped by the ethos, values, and practices of the corporate culture, adding to the impersonality of the hospital milieu. At the same time, care and compassion are professed in facsimile by impersonal framed statements posted on the walls of the hospitals.

Another factor in the erosion of the professionalism of medicine has been the rise of feminism and its questioning of so-called patriarchal ideals and practices. There has been criticism of medicine's most important claim, namely, that its therapies are soundly based on knowledge that is scientifically based and garnered through meticulous observation and critical experiment; for they point out that the gender discrimination of many large-scale studies invalidates the general applicability of the results to women. The medical practices of the male-dominated "hi-tech" specialty of obstetrics and gynaecology have been criticized as being too technically oriented; and they have supported the emergence of a free-standing midwifery profession—an exact counterpoise to the emergence of the male-midwife movement of the eighteenth century. Other healthcare professions, particularly nursing, question and criticize the professional hegemony and dominance of medicine. The modern nursing profession defines its own knowledge base, educational mandate, and evaluation; creates its own nursing management of patients, complementing those of medicine; and does not regard itself as subservient to medicine but as separate, different, and equal.[51]

Today, the exclusivity of medical knowledge can no longer be taken as given. The diffusion of technical medical knowledge beyond the confines of a select group and the creation of that knowledge by others than formally recognized medical practitioners, e.g., biochemists and other scientists, together with the rise of consumerism has also had an impact of the authority of the profession. Every newspaper, magazine, and television station has a health care commentator and offers advice about health and the management of diseases. Specialized support groups offer not only support but also make available the latest findings of research and practice within their particular area of interest. The net result is not only to make the patient an informed consumer, but also to restore the imbalance in the power relation between doctor and patient.

The replacement of the ethical basis of medicine from its base as a physician-formulated ethic with a voluntary commitment to the patient's interest to the obligatory supremacy of patient rights and entitlements, a transformation both recent and revolutionary, has created an adversarial basis to the doctor-patient relationship, a *caveat-emptor* approach replacing trust, confidence, and commitment. Sociologists such as Eliot Freidson and lay critics such as Ivan Illich have assailed the claims of the profession for the primacy of patient interest, for service unencumbered by selfish interest.[52]

The erosion of the supremacy of science as the dominant explanatory mechanism has also had its impact on the credibility of medicine and doctors,[53] while the revelations of scientific fraud,[54] scientific exploitation of the helpless during the Cold War era,[55] systematic involvement in torture[56] and mass extermination,[57] and the exposure of physician sexual abuse as well as venality have eroded the image of the profession as honourable and dedicated to the primacy of patient interest.

Perspectives on Professionalism

The drive towards the modern professionalism of medicine arose in the era of *laissez-faire* economics and cut across the unfettered expression of market freedom. Emile Durkheim (1858–1917) suggested that professions were a means of moral renewal within an otherwise anomic society, for they fostered a sense of obligation and order rather than individualistic expression.[58] Talcott Parsons also emphasized that professions served the common good with their community-orientation as opposed to the self-orientation of business occupations.[59]

The medical monopoly is threatened by the emergence of alternative therapies as well as by the demand of other healthcare practitioners to act as "gatekeepers" to the health care system.

The Ethos of the Age

In this day and age, characterized by the primacy of self-interest and dominated by the ideology and economic imperialism of the market, the dominant social paradigm—in direct contradiction to the statement of our Lord and Master—is that "a man's life does consist in the abundance of things that he or she possesses" (cf. Luke 12:15). If the pursuit of wealth is the main reason for undertaking any enterprise, whether it be profession, business, athletic endeavour, and even those of intimacy such as marriage (as history will attest), then the resultant values and behaviours will be radically different from those obtaining when the enterprise is undertaken for its own sake and interest or for some larger goal of service.[60]

The current emphasis on the exclusively contractual nature of all relationships, with the corresponding reliance upon written codes and formally expressed rights, might seem to be the pinnacle of the evolution of a democratic society. However, any sense of obligation beyond the immediate duty to hand is effectively removed and pre-

cludes any sense of grace or works of supererogation (Latin, *rogare*—
"to ask") in all relationships between persons, and fosters a wariness,
even suspicion of others. The assumption that personal and material
self-interest of the doctor dominates the relationship between doctor
and patient rather than a beneficent commitment to patient interest
and welfare has transformed the climate in which medicine is practised from one characterized by trust to one shaped by suspicion,
from genuine relationship to a commercialism, from a clinical realis-
tic medicine to a defensive medicine governed by medical self-
protection against legal threat rather than by diagnostic necessity or
acumen.

If we believe that the unrestrained pursuit of private gain is the
best means by which a public gain might possibly be developed, arising as an unintended by-product, then we should not be surprised
that public trust is replaced by a corrosive, and yet protective, cynicism of all professional and public activities. If morality, personal
behaviour, and professional activity can be promulgated by legislation, defined by law, controlled by bureaucratic supervision, while
simultaneously exploited by unscrupulous manipulation, why
should one be a person of integrity, compassion, justice, and honour? The prevalence and dominance of such attitudes will, to borrow
the phrases written during the turmoil of the English Civil War
(1642–1658) by that arch-sceptic, Thomas Hobbes (1568–1679), ensure that life will again become "solitary, poor, nasty, brutish, and
short" as each pursues their private interest, "a condition of war of
everyone against everyone."[61]

Responses of the Christian

Today, the medical practitioner is being obliged to serve two masters,
that is, to practise medicine with a divided loyalty where the primacy
of patient interest is being eroded by other interests: those of society,
of the HMO, and of the managed care organization. To continue
the dominical quotation, "he will hold to the one, and despise the
other." (Mt 6:24 KJV). All too often, doctors are vilified as being venal, exploitative, and of doubtful competence. More than ever, even
more so than in the days of Gregory and Percival, doctors must be
men and women of virtue, marked by their integrity, honesty, truth-
fulness, faithfulness, and compassion as well as their competence.

The Transformed Mind

As Christian doctors, we must not be squeezed into the patterns, values, and behaviours of this age—with its pursuit of power, wealth, and celebrity—and neither must we adopt the mechanistic perceptions, attitudes, and goals of medicine in this postmodern era. "Therefore, I urge you, brothers, in view of God's mercy, to offer your bodies as living sacrifices, holy and pleasing to God—this is your spiritual [alternate reading: reasonable] act of worship. Do not conform any longer to the pattern of this world, but be transformed by the renewing of your mind. Then you will be able to test and approve what God's will is—his good, pleasing and perfect will" (Rom 12:1-2).

The Transformed Attitude

As Christian doctors, we need more than ever to emphasise the servant character, not only of our faith, but also of the profession, with a commitment to care for the patient as the first obligation. "Your attitude should be the same as that of Jesus Christ: Who, being in very nature God, did not consider equality with God something to be grasped, but made himself nothing, taking the very nature of a servant . . ." (Phil 2:5-7).

The Transforming Action

We need to be alongside the patient, to meet with them as persons, to be where they are in their need, and to exhibit the touch of compassion and therapy rather than be only the detached and impersonal observers of the objectivized patient, acting as mere mechanics of the diseased body. "A Samaritan as he travelled, came where the man was; and when he saw him, he took pity on him. He went to him, and bandaged his wounds, pouring on oil and wine . . ." (cf. Lk 10:30-36).

Notes

1   H. Perkins, *The Rise of Professional Society: England since 1880* (London: Routledge, 1989), 2–3.

2   H. Perkins, *The Origins of Modern English Society, 1780–1880* (Toronto: University of Toronto Press, 1972), 24.

3   T. Jefferson, "Original Draft for the Declaration of Independence," in *The Con-*

cise *Oxford Dictionary of Quotations* (Oxford University Press, 1964), 113.

4   I. Kant, *Groundwork of a Metaphysic of Morals*, trans. H. J. Paton (New York: Harper & Row, Harper Torchbooks, 1956), 30.

5   E. H. Hunt, *British Labour History, 1815–1914* (London: Wiedenfeld and Nicholson, 1985), 14.

6   P. A. Gregg, *Social and Economic History of Britain, 1760–1950* (London: George Harrap & Co., 1952), 30.

7   W. Wordsworth, "The Excursion," Book VIII, *The Parsonage*, lines 180–85, in *The Poetical Works of William Wordsworth*, ed. T. Hutchinson (Oxford: Humphrey Milford Press, 1920), 877.

8   E. H. Phelps Brown and S. V. Hopkins, "Seven Centuries of the Prices of Consumables Compared with Builders' Wage Rates," *Economica 1956*, quoted in P. Deane, *The First Industrial Revolution*, 2nd ed. (Cambridge: Cambridge University Press, 1979), 31–32.

9   E. Chadwick, *Report on the Sanitary Condition of the Labouring Population of Great Britain* (London: Poor Law Commission, 1842; reprinted Edinburgh, Edinburgh University Press, 1965), 157, excerpted in D. J. Rothman, S. Marcus, and S. A. Kiceluk, eds., *Medicine and Western Civilization* (New Brunswick, N.J.: Rutgers University Press, 1995), 217–239.

10 D. Porter, "Public Health," in *Companion Encyclopaedia of the History of Medicine*, eds. W. F. Bynum and R. Porter, 2 vols. (London: Routledge, 1993), 2:1242.

11 A. Pope, *Essay on Man*, Epistle I, Part X, lines 289–95, in *Collected Poems of Alexander Pope*, ed. Bonamee Dobry (New York: Dutton, Everyman's Library Edition, 1963), 189.

12 A. Pope, *Moral Essays*, Epistle IV, "To Richard Boyle, Earl of Burlington," lines 165–72, in *Collected Poems*, 251.

13 M. Hovell, *The Chartist Movement*, ed. T. F. Tout, 3rd ed. (Manchester, England: University of Manchester Press, 1966), 174–90.

14 J. W. Willcock, *The Laws Relating to the Medical Profession* (1830), 30, quoted in S. W. F. Holloway, "Medical Education in England, 1830–1858," *History* 49, no. 167 (1964): 299–324, 306.

15 Holloway, "Medical Education in England," 299–306.

16 I. Loudin, *Medical Care and the General Practitioner, 1750–1850* (Oxford: Clarendon Press, 1986), 129.

17 Sir Anthony Carlisle, hospital surgeon, testimony, *British House of Commons Select Committee of Medical Education, 1834* (602-ii), xiii, part ii, Q 5809-12, (), 125-6.

18 B. Rush, "The Vices and Virtues of Physicians," in *Selected Writings of Benjamin Rush*, ed. Dagobert D. Runes (New York: Philosophical Library, 1946), quoted in D. J. Rothman, S. Marcus, and S. A. Kiceluk, eds., *Medicine and Western Civilization*, (New Brunswick, N.J.: Rutgers University Press, 1995), 278–81.

19 G. Smith and A. Munro, *History of the Bristol Royal Infirmary* (Bristol: J. W. Ar-

rowsmith, 1917), 24, 97.

[20] I. Waddington, The Medical Profession in the Industrial Revolution (Dublin: Gill & Macmillan Humanities Press, 1984), 159–62.

[21] Loudin, Medical Care, 250–51. James Handey of Upper Stamford St., London, "The First to Try, and Successfully, the Legality of Charges for Visits From General Practitioners," Medical Directory (1848). See also T. Wakley, Lancet 1 (1829–30): 539; "Remuneration of General Practitioners," London Medical Gazette (1830): 665–7.

[22] D. Porter and R. Porter, Patient's Progress: Doctors and Doctoring in Eighteenth-Century England (Palo Alto, Calif.: Stanford University Press, 1989), 18–27.

[23] E. Harrison, Remarks on the Ineffective State of the Practice of Physic in Great Britain, with Proposals for Its Future Regulation and Improvement (London: R. Bickerstaff, 1806), 1–2, 38–9.

[24] Holloway, "Medical Education in England," 299–324.

[25] C. Lawrence, "William Buchan: Medicine Laid Open," Medical History, 14 (1975): 19–35. C. Rosenberg, "Medical Text and Medical Context: Explaining Willam Buchan's 'Domestic Medicine'," Bull Hist Med 62 (1983): 22–4.

[26] J. Wesley, "Primitive Physic (1755)," in John Wesley's Book of Old Fashioned Cures and Remedies, ed. W. H. Paynter (Plymouth, England: Parade Printing Works, 1958).

[27] T. Turner, The Diary of Thomas Turner, 1754–1756, ed. D. Vaisey (Oxford: Oxford University Press, 1984).

[28] N. D. Jewson, "Medical Knowledge and the Patronage System in Eighteenth-Century England," Sociology 8 (1974): 369–857.

[29] G. Miller, The Introduction of Inoculation for Smallpox in England and France (London: Oxford University Press, 1957).

[30] Jewson, "Medical Knowledge," 369–857.

[31] I. Waddington, The Medical Profession, 186–90.

[32] M. W. Flinn, British Population Growth, 1700–1850 (London: MacMillan, 1970); E. J. Evans, The Forging of the Modern State: Early Industrial Britain, 1783–1870 (London: Longman, 1987), 404–7.

[33] J. Gregory, Lectures on the Duties and Qualifications of a Physician (London: W. Stahan & T. Cadell, 1772), Lecture 4, 5.

[34] Ibid., 38.

[35] Ibid., 39–40.

[36] Ibid., 38.

[37] T. Percival, Medical Ethics, Or, a Code of Institutions and Precepts Adapted to the Professional Conduct of Physicians and Surgeons (1803; Birmingham, Alabama: The Classics of Medicine Library, Gryphon editions, 1985), 2; G. L. Higgins, "Professionalism: Ethics vs Etiquette," Canad Fam Phys 36 (1990): 1946–48.

[38] Percival, viii–ix.

39 R. M. Kerrison, *An Inquiry into the Present State of the Medical Profession in England* (London: Longman, Hurst, Rees et al., 1814), 29–30.

40 W. O. Porter, *Medical Science and Ethicks: An Introductory Lecture* (Bristol: W. Strong, 1837), quoted in Waddington, *The Medical Profession*, 161.

41 Ibid.

42 S. W. F. Holloway, "The Apothecaries' Act 1815: A Reinterpretation. Part 2: The Consequences of the Act," *Medical History* 10, no. 3 (1966): 221–36.

43 F. F. Cartwright, *A Social History of Medicine* (London: Longmans, Hurst, Rees et al., 1977), 53.

44 Loudin, *Medical Care*, 169–70.

45 Cartwright, *A Social History of Medicine*, 56.

46 I. Waddington, "The Movement towards the Professionalisation of Medicine," *Brit Med J* 30, no. 2 (1990): 688–90.

47 W. F. Bynum, *Science and the Practice of Medicine in the Nineteenth Century.* (Cambridge: Cambridge University Press, 1995), 180.

48 Waddington, "The Movement," 688–90.

49 E. Shorter, *Bedside Manners: The Troubled History of Doctors and Patients* (New York: Simon & Schuster, 1985), 17–25.

50 J. L. Graner, "The Primary Care Crisis: The Degradation of the Modern Physician from Artist to Labourer," *Humane Medicine* 7, no. 3 (1991): 189–194.

51 J. L. Storch, "Division of Labour in Health Care: Pragmatics and Ethics," *Humane Medicine* 10, no. 4 (1994): 262–69.

52 Eliot Freidson has studied the American medical profession intensively and published a number of books e.g., *Professional Dominance: The Social Structure of Medical Care* (Chicago: Aldine, 1970); *Profession of Medicine: A Study of the Sociology of Applied Knowledge* (Chicago: University of Chicago Press, 1970, 1988); *Medical Work in America: Essays on Health Care* (New Haven, Conn.: Yale University Press, 1989); *Professionalism Reborn: Theory, Prophecy and Policy* (Chicago: University of Chicago Press, 1994); and with co-author J. Lorber, *Medical Men and Their Work: A Sociological Reader* (Chicago: AldineAtherton, 1972); I. Illich, *Medical Nemesis: The Expropiation of Health* (Toronto: McClelland & Stewart, 1975).

53 D. E. Chubin and E. W. Chu, eds., *Science off the Pedestal: Social Perspectives on Science and Technology* (Belmont, Calif.: Wadsworth Publishing, 1989).

54 H. K. Beecher, "Ethics and Clinical Research," *New Eng J Med* 274 (1966): 1354–60; W. Broad and N. Wade, *Betrayers of the Truth; Fraud and Deceit in the Halls of Science* (New York: Simon & Schuster, 1982); A. Kohn, *False Prophets: Fraud and Error in Science and Medicine* (Oxford: Blackwell, 1986).

55 W. Marston, "Friendly Fire: Radiation Victims of the Cold War," *The Sciences* 34, no. 2 (1994): 48.

56 British Medical Association Report of a Working Party, *Medicine Betrayed: The Participation of Doctors in Human Rights Abuses* (London: British Medical Associa-

tion, 1992); V. Marange, Amnesty International French Medical Commission, *Doctors and Torture: Collaboration or Resistance?*, intro. C. Glass, trans. A. Andrews (London: Bellew Publishing Co., 1989).

57 M. H. Kater, *Doctors Under Hitler* (Chapel Hill, N.C.: University of North Carolina Press, 1989); R. J. Lifton, *The Nazi Doctors: Medical Killing and the Psychology of Genocide* (New York: Basic Books, 1986).

58 E. Durkhein, *Professional Ethics and Civic Morals*, trans. C. Brookfield, foreward by B. S. Turner, 2nd ed. (London: Routledge, 1992).

59 Talcott Parsons, "The Professions and Social Structure," in *Essays in Sociological Theory*, rev. ed. (Glencoe, Ill.: Free Press, 1954).

60 B. Schwarz, *The Battle for Human Nature: Science, Morality and Modern Life* (New York: W. W. Norton, 1986), 247–80.

61 T. Hobbes, *Leviathan*, part I, ch. 13, ed. C. B. Macpherson (Markham, Ont.: Penguin Books, 1988), 185–86.

James Houston

These Three Remain: Faith, Hope, Love

I t is perhaps in medicine, in bioethics, and in the social sciences generally, where Christians feel most marginalized. Why? Is it not because in every way possible the spiritual nature of Man is being denied, to permit the study of Man to be recognized as "scientific" as possible? Faith then is substituted by cognitive certainty. Is it not also, because the nature of Man is being grounded in this world only, in this present existence, where cause and effect are empirically defined and controlled, so that *telos* is mechanical, not divine? Hope then, is substituted by pragmatism, infinitude by the finite, God by self-realization. Is it not also, because secularism and scientism are a "flight from tenderness" and thus stand in antithesis to the personal and the religious, which seek above all to experience the love of God? Love then, is substituted by control, the quest for power, not for openness of "being-for-the-other." Thus a love-less society becomes a reductionist society, where abortion, euthanasia, and every other anti-human posture in between life and death are not only tolerated but actually advocated.

No wonder Christian professionals, operating out of such a Technological Society, feel increasingly pressurized and marginalized. For it is becoming an increasingly hostile environment, no longer accepting of the Christian values that undergirded the "take-off" that launched the modern world. We live then in an age of supreme apostasy, with the deliberate rejection of those very elements of the Reformation that made modern society a possibility after the sixteenth century—the empirical awareness of an intelligible cosmos, whose rationality was as dependable as its Creator was. It upheld an anthropology that reflected the *imago Dei*, giving dignity, responsibility, and stewardship to Man within the created order, both to seek God and to understand within the mandate of true science. No other religion provided that. Nor were the motives for thrift in commerce, diligence in industry, care and compassion in medicine, education and nurture of youth, found other than in Christianity to provided infrastructures for the possibilities of the modern world. Secularism today shoots itself in the foot—indeed, in the heart!

You have come to this Conference, then, to encourage one another, Christians witnessing the death of Christendom, but thank God, not the loss of Christ. For as we encourage one another, and build one another up, as Paul exhorted the Thessalonians to do, Christ becomes ever more central to each one of us. Yet we do not understand how easy it is to become demoralized, disillusioned perhaps, by the trends of reductionism operative in contemporary professionalism—for are we not being forced back behind Constantine and Christendom to the minority situation of the early Christians, to the position of simply being witnesses, like candles in an all encompassing darkness—a dark age indeed.

I share this deep sense of marginalization with you, first in my professional life as an Oxford Don, then in the experiment of Regent College, and then still further as engaged in a prophetic posture within the remnants of Christendom. Yet it is a posture with its dangers of self-concern and self-isolation, unless we also see the bigger picture of viewing human existence meta-anthropologically, as Man before God; so that civilization, ancient and modern are seen in the light of biblical meta-history, and human behaviour is likewise seen in terms of meta-ethics, of Man made in the image and likeness of God, creatively and redemptively so.

However, the enculturation of divine revelation has distorted the central image of Christ throughout the last two millennia. The lingering influence of classical culture and its underlying Stoic assumptions still entwine the theological graces of faith, hope, and love with the so-called "cardinal virtues" of prudence, justice, fortitude, and temperance. This creates a Pelagian admixture of "God helps those who help themselves," of a life of faith with a virtuous life. But what happens when postmodernist philosophers reject the metaphysical dimension of reality? Then we have classical humanists like Iris

Murdoch, *Metaphysics as a Guide to Morals* (1992), or Alasdair McIntyre, *After Virtue* (1981), who despair of the impending dissolution of the Stoic life of virtue.

So what is the Christian response? Positively, we can celebrate: "Thank goodness, Christendom is over." Like Søren Kierkegaard, we can feel freer when the ideational and the ideological are no longer substitutes for personal encounter with God. Or like Benjamin Disraeli's epigram in his novels: "Read no history; nothing but biography, for that is life without theory." The claims of the actual, rather than theory, is the excitement we feel about Shakespeare. Even more so, the realm of the actual, the particular, the personal, is the sphere of Christian faith. Meanwhile, moralists who make a science out of human behaviour still endlessly quarrel among themselves: which comes first, prudence, i.e., "know-how," or justice, i.e., "do to others what you want done to yourself"? Thus, moralists tend to negate other prescriptions, rather than affirm what to be and do, because behaviour is treated too anthropocentrically.

Instead, this Conference has affirmed that "these three remain: faith, hope, love." Indeed, this is more than an epigram. These are the "three imperishables" of Christian reality in a world rife with illusion and confusion. Together they embrace the whole of Christian existence and experience, as lived out by each individual Christian in corporate solidarity with all other Christians through time and space. It is evident in Paul's epistles that he lived fully aware of the Stoics' moral realm of the virtuous life. But he never refers to the cardinal virtues, not even when he catalogues the vices of the pagan world, and gives a list of the fruit of the Spirit (Gal 5:22-23). His punctuation may well have been "the fruit of the Spirit is love," followed then by what is descriptive of love's expressions, divinely as the gifts of love, joy, peace; socially as patience, kindness, goodness; and personally as faithfulness, gentleness, and self-control.

Likewise in 1 Corinthians 13, faith and hope are related to this hymn that celebrates the excellence and primacy of divine love. For faith is the assurance given by God's love and hope rests and presses forward in the love of God. That is why "the greatest of these is love." Each is inter-related and inter-dependent upon the others, as expressive of God's very Being. Faith has Christ as it hopes in Christ, and loves through Christ. He is the Foundation that is laid, beside which there is no other (1 Cor 3:11).

Faith then is central to the life and teaching of the apostle Paul. "The life I now live in the flesh, I live by the faith of the Son of God" (Gal 2:20 RSV). Well do I remember, when I realized that I did not live by *my* faith, but rather lived by the benefits of Christ's faithfulness, who invites us to share in the filial trust of the Son in the Father, through the Holy Spirit. As Pascal, Kierkegaard, and many other thoughtful saints have pointed out, the very structure of our human existence cries out for faith-in-the-Other. For we literally cannot enter life, live as a child, as a growing adult, as a *person*, without basic trust in another's trustworthiness. The theologian Hans Urs von Balthasar sees the babe's first recognition of the mother's smile with a responsive smile as the first miraculous awakening into human relatedness of the "I" created in responsivity to the "Thou." So the Christian too, is awakened to the basic trustworthiness of God in his Word, to go on living by "every word that proceeds from the mouth of God." It is now, at the end of Christendom, that Christians are again being called out to witness to the faith of the Gospel, indeed, to witness unto death if necessary, before an unbelieving, hostile world. So Christian doctors, nurses, and many other helping professionals may need to be prepared to sacrifice careers, ambitions, and much else, if called upon, in order to remain faithful witnesses.

Hope is an inseparable reality of Christian faith. Karl Barth speaks of the "great" and of the "little hope" of the Christian, that is the prospect of eternal life that is also experienced daily in ordinary life. So hopefulness is the life-style of the Christian. This is the antidote to so much of the quiet despair of many desperate moderns who live under a secular canopy of reductionism, that knows only materialism, rationalism, pragmatism, and indeed many other -isms, as idols in place of God. Many ethical issues would not be so poignant and so problematic, were there more hope in our society. But the loss of transcendent vision, substituted by technical *telos* as mechanical cause and effect, trivializes our culture in such meaningless ways. If guilt blocks our past in despair, presumption may also block our future in pride. Hence the present is the realm of boredom for many in our world today, blocked backward by guilt, blocked forward by presumption.

But for the Christian, the last word is the primacy and supremacy of love, as Paul reminds us in his great celebration of *agape* in 1 Corinthians 13. Love occupies the supreme place in heaven, for "God is love." It should also occupy then the central place in the life of the Christian. So where faith looks back to Calvary, to free us from our past inheritance of sin; and hope looks forward to free us from anxiety; love expands and enriches the present consciousness of the Christian, to see the vastness of the horizon before each worshipper of our loving God. Indeed, God's love is the real substance of faith and hope.

What then does God's love really mean to you and me? It means the transformation of our entirely creaturely existence, for "God's love is shed abroad in our hearts by the Holy Spirit." Only lovers know love, and so in Victorian prudery, Edward Coswall, afraid to offend his audience, mis-translated Bernard of Clairvaux's great hymn as:

The love of Jesus, what it is

None but His loved ones know.

While Bernard had really said:

The love of Jesus, what it is,

None but His *lovers* know.

We live largely by our loves, and they define us. Beyond the love of our professions, may our loves ever and always be determined by the transcendence of the love of God.